SHAPING OUR SELVES

SHAPING OUR SELVES

On Technology, Flourishing, and a Habit of Thinking

Erik Parens

OXFORD
UNIVERSITY PRESS

OXFORD

UNIVERSITY PRESS

Oxford University Press is a department of the University of Oxford.
It furthers the University's objective of excellence in research,
scholarship, and education by publishing worldwide.

Oxford   New York
Auckland   Cape Town   Dar es Salaam   Hong Kong   Karachi
Kuala Lumpur   Madrid   Melbourne   Mexico City   Nairobi
New Delhi   Shanghai   Taipei   Toronto

With offices in
Argentina   Austria   Brazil   Chile   Czech Republic   France   Greece
Guatemala   Hungary   Italy   Japan   Poland   Portugal   Singapore
South Korea   Switzerland   Thailand   Turkey   Ukraine   Vietnam

Oxford is a registered trademark of Oxford University Press
in the UK and certain other countries.

Published in the United States of America by
Oxford University Press
198 Madison Avenue, New York, NY 10016

© Oxford University Press 2015

First issued as an Oxford University Press paperback, 2016

All rights reserved. No part of this publication may be reproduced, stored in
a retrieval system, or transmitted, in any form or by any means, without the prior
permission in writing of Oxford University Press, or as expressly permitted by law,
by license, or under terms agreed with the appropriate reproduction rights organization.
Inquiries concerning reproduction outside the scope of the above should be sent to the
Rights Department, Oxford University Press, at the address above.

You must not circulate this work in any other form
and you must impose this same condition on any acquirer.

Library of Congress Cataloging-in-Publication Data
Parens, Erik, 1957– author.
Shaping our selves : on technology, flourishing, and a habit of thinking / Erik Parens.
p. ; cm.
ISBN 978-0-19-021174-5 (hardcover); 978-0-19-064589-2 (paperback)
I. Title.
[DNLM: 1. Bioethical Issues.   2. Body Image.   3. Biomedical Technology— ethics.
4. Reconstructive Surgical Procedures—ethics.   5. Social Perception.   WB 60]
R725.5
174.2′97952—dc23
2014015236

"If you want the truth to stand clear before you, never be for or against. The struggle between 'for' and 'against' is the mind's worst disease."

—The words of a Buddhist teacher

"Which Side Are You On?"

—The title of a civil rights song

CONTENTS

ACKNOWLEDGMENTS

For help in creating this book, I am deeply grateful to many people. Josephine Johnston shared with me an ongoing conversation about the book's central issues, while we drove to and from, and while we were at, our shared place of work, The Hastings Center. Josie patiently read and generously commented on the first draft, as did David Wasserman. Nathan Kravis, Barry Hoffmaster, and Saskia Nagel all read a second draft, and all offered extensive and insightful comments. In the fall of 2012, I had the good fortune of visiting the Ethics Institute of Utrecht University (in the Netherlands) for a week, and I received still more helpful suggestions from Joel Anderson, Ineke Bolt, Marcus Duwell, Caroline Harnacke, and Maartje Schermer. Lisa Hedley, Laura Mauldin, and Maya Sabatello shared their insights regarding individual chapters, and I have had the great benefit of ongoing conversation with all of my other colleagues at The Hastings Center, in particular Gregory Kaebnick.

I am also grateful to the students in my seminars in the Science, Technology, and Society Programs at Vassar College and at Sarah

ACKNOWLEDGMENTS

Lawrence. Sitting in a seminar room, talking about a text, with 15 or 20 smart, insightful, well-prepared students has been one of my life's great pleasures thus far. I thank those students, and a long line of terrific research assistants at the Center, including, several years ago, Jacob Moses and, most recently, Naomi Scheinerman.

My editor at Oxford University Press, Lucy Randall, has, from the beginning, offered kind encouragement, keen insight, and clear suggestions. Lucy also recruited two peer reviewers, whose identities I have since learned; thanks, too, to Jackie Leach Scully and to Ilina Singh. This book is better than it would have been, had they not given their time to offer criticisms and suggestions.

I am also indebted to the generous scholars I had the chance to work with on projects that I have led or co-led at The Hastings Center, including two funded by the National Endowment for the Humanities ("On the Prospect of Technologies Aimed at the Enhancement of Human Capacities" and "Surgically Shaping Children"); three funded by the National Institutes of Health ("Prenatal Testing for Genetic Disability," "Crafting Tools for Public Conversation about Behavioral Genetics," and "Pharmacological Treatment of Behavioral Disturbances in Children: Engaging the Controversies"); and one funded by the Dana Foundation ("Interpreting Neuroimages: Interdisciplinary Engagement with the Complexities"). Also of great benefit was working with the scholars on The Hastings Center's project "Ethical Issues in Synthetic Biology," which was funded by the Alfred P. Sloan Foundation.

It has been an extraordinary privilege to receive scarce grant dollars to do work that promises, not to improve anybody's health or financial portfolio, but to explore questions about the meaning of advances in science, medicine, and technology. I am grateful to Daniel Callahan and Willard Gaylin for having had the vision to create an institution for asking such questions, and I am equally grateful to The Hastings Center's President, Millie Solomon, and to our remarkable board of directors for their unstinting commitment to bringing Dan and Will's vision forward.

Most of all, I thank my wife, Andrea Kott, whose generosity, patience, and love fill me with gratitude. It has been a long, good time now that we have shared the challenge, and great joy, of trying to shape our children, Sophie and Ben, and also trying to let them unfold in their own ways.

Last, I gratefully acknowledge that in this book I draw on parts of articles I have published before. Chapter 1 draws on "Is Better Always Good? The Enhancement Project," *Hastings Center Report* 28, no. 1 (1998): S1–S20. Chapter 3 draws on both "Authenticity and Ambivalence: Toward Understanding the Enhancement Debate," *Hastings Center Report* 35, no. 3 (2005): 34–41, and "Toward a More Fruitful Debate about Human Enhancement," in *Human Enhancement*, ed. Julian Savulescu and Nick Bostrom (Oxford: Oxford University Press, 2009), 181–98. Chapter 4 draws on "Creativity, Gratitude, and the Enhancement Debate," in *Neuroethics in the 21st Century*, ed. Judith Illes (Oxford: Oxford University Press, 2005), 75–86. Chapter 5 draws on both "On Good and Bad Forms of Medicalization," *Bioethics* 27, no. 1 (2013): 28–35, and "The Ethics of Memory Blunting and the Narcissism of Small Differences," *Neuroethics* 3, no. 2 (2010): 99–107.

Introduction

I'm not sure I ever heard the term *bioethics* before 1992, when the philosopher Daniel Callahan hired me to be his research assistant at the world's first bioethics research institute, The Hastings Center. As the cofounder and then president of the Center, Callahan was apparently one of the only employers in the country impressed by my PhD from an unusual and eccentric program at the University of Chicago called the Committee on Social Thought. Rightly, Callahan thought that the Committee attracted faculty and students like him: people somewhat oblivious to traditional academic borders, but powerfully drawn to the big, old questions about the meaning of being human and about how we ought to live—people who believe that asking those questions can itself be an integral part of living well and that asking them together can even, incrementally, contribute to promoting the flourishing of ever more human beings.

When I was a student at the Committee in the 1980s, I didn't study bioethics. I studied an idiosyncratic mix of ancient Greek philosophy and poetry, as well as 19th- and 20th-century philosophy and psychology, and I wrote a dissertation about the relationship between Nietzsche's politics and his philosophy of nature. Because, when I graduated from the Committee in the late 1980s, there wasn't a big market for people who followed their own intellectual noses, I had to accept a string of one- and two-year teaching posts. In 1992, however, my dissertation advisor, Leon Kass—the most wonderful and important of the many wonderful and important teachers I had at the University of Chicago—mentioned that Daniel Callahan was looking to make a junior hire at The Hastings Center. When I was a student at the Committee, Kass was not yet known internationally as a staunch and sometimes strident critic of emerging biotechnologies, nor had he yet been named the chair of George W. Bush's President's Council on Bioethics. He had, however, been a founding fellow of The Hastings Center, and when he wrote to Callahan on my behalf, Callahan took his letter seriously.

So overnight, by accepting a job at The Hastings Center, I went from being an itinerant professor of the humanities to being a "bioethicist." From the start, part of my job was opining to reporters on bioethical issues of the day. Should a health care system use scarce resources to separate conjoined twins? Should physicians be permitted to grant patient requests for assisted suicide? Should prospective parents be permitted to select embryos for traits they desire? And so forth.

One day I was being interviewed by Rick Weiss, who then was a reporter at the *Washington Post*, and whom I had grown to like and respect very much. I found myself once again asking him not to refer to me in his story as a bioethicist. I explained that, no, he shouldn't call me a philosopher, because that refers to someone with a PhD from a philosophy department, and that he also shouldn't call me a "thinker," because that sounds pretentious, and "gadfly" is both obscure and grandiose. "Well," Weiss asked, "what *should* I call you?" After I granted that I didn't have a good alternative, he exasperatedly offered help: "Maybe I should call you a wizard—like the one in Oz who sits behind the curtain, understands all, and can solve everyone's problems!"

Many years later, I still dislike being called a bioethicist, because I fear that after that label trails the fantasy that bioethical wizards exist—beings who, presumably due to their genetic endowment or superior parents or education or powers of reasoning, do understand all and who therefore have moral expertise, which enables them to know better than others what we as individuals and as a society ought to do with regard to advances in bio-techno-science. I worry that the bioethicist label can feed the idea that, just like you go to a lawyer for an expert answer to a legal question, or to a mechanic for an answer about your car, or to a neurologist for an answer about your brain, you go to a bioethicist for an expert answer to your bioethical question.

Here's the problem. The lawyer knows what you want and can tell you if current laws will likely support your effort to get it. The mechanic and the neurologist also know what you want, and if they can't fix your problem, usually they can at least name it. You, the lawyer, the mechanic, and the neurologist can agree about what you want and about how to achieve it. Nobody asks, Should I want to win this case? or How do we know when my car is working well? or What attitude ought my neurosurgeon adopt toward the tumor growing in my brain? In those cases, we already agree about the desirability or goodness of the purpose that we hope the professional will help us achieve.

But with the sorts of bioethical questions that most capture my attention, what's at issue is precisely what our purpose or aim should be. These are the big questions about the meaning of being human and about how we ought to live: questions about the nature of persons and what makes them truly flourish, about the nature of the various means we use to pursue our flourishing, about what if anything we owe our fellow citizens when we seek our flourishing, and so forth. Such questions—which I will gather under the label of "meaning questions"—do not admit of expert or crisp or final answers. They demand more conversation.

None of this is to say that people referred to as bioethicists never have any answers. In chapter 1, I explain a way in which they can and do. Here I'm simply emphasizing that there are no crisp, final, expert answers to the sorts of meaning questions I find most engaging and that are at stake in the debates I explore in this book. These are the debates concerning the use of technologies like surgery, pharmacology, and genetics to shape ourselves and our children. I'm suggesting that these debates about technologically shaping our selves are a wonderful opportunity to appreciate the difference between questions for which we should expect crisp answers, and questions for which we should instead expect a long, productive-albeit-never-finished conversation. Indeed, my primary aim in this book is to articulate a habit of thinking about those meaning questions. My secondary aim is to show how such a habit of thinking can help promote at least one sort of action: the act of choosing whether to use a technology to shape ourselves or our children.

THE PLAN

When I say that this book's primary aim is to articulate a habit of thinking about meaning questions, it may sound like I plan to stray far from the world of lived experience. Actually, I am deeply interested in the extent to which our thinking grows out of our experience. In particular, I am interested in the extent to which, for better and for worse, our ethical stances and conclusions are shaped by more than reason alone. I am interested in how they are shaped by forces including our histories and feelings—where, with the term *feelings*, I refer to that huge class of phenomena, including emotions and intuitions, to which we do not consciously reason our way. In chapter 1, "Seeing from Somewhere in Particular," I need to say a bit about my own history leading up to, and my own feelings regarding, the subset of debates about technologically shaping our selves that I consider at greatest length in this book: the debates concerning the "enhancement" of human traits and capacities. In this chapter I suggest that we should set aside the pleasure associated with arguing *for* or *against* enhancement, so that we can benefit from the insights associated with thinking *about* enhancement—about the meaning of enhancement.

In chapter 2, "Embracing Binocularity," I explain what I mean when I say that our habit of thinking and, ultimately, acting would be better if it were more "binocular." A more binocular habit of thinking assumes that, much as we achieve visual depth perception by integrating the slightly different information that our two eyes give us, we can aspire to achieve depth of intellectual understanding by integrating the greatly different insights that myriad pairs of conceptual lenses give us. In this chapter I introduce one of the most prominent of those pairs that appears throughout these debates: through one lens we see our selves as subjects who have the experience of choosing freely, and through the other we see our selves as objects, whose behaviors are determined by a staggeringly complex array of biological and social forces, which interact over time. A more binocular approach to thinking accepts the energy-consuming work of oscillating between the insights afforded by the subject and object lenses. Such an approach also accepts that, though, in principle, using two conceptual lenses at once would facilitate perfect intellectual depth perception, in practice, we aren't built for using two at once. That is, I suggest that we should aspire to more binocular thinking, and we should accept that perfectly binocular thinking isn't achievable.

A more binocular approach doesn't only aspire to oscillate between the apparently opposing insights at work in distinctions like the one between object and subject. As I intend to signal with the book's two epigraphs, a more binocular approach also aspires to embrace the tension between the demands made on us by activities like thinking and acting. In the context of the activity I think most about in this book—choosing whether to request or refuse a technological intervention—I will not only suggest that perfectly binocular thinking is humanly impossible, but also acknowledge the way in which more binocular thinking can become ethically undesirable. That is, more binocular thinking becomes ethically undesirable if it becomes an excuse for inaction. There comes a point in the process of choosing where the oscillation between lenses has to stop. I will hold out the hope that, even if choosing whether to use a technological intervention requires us to stop the sort of oscillation that more binocular thinking requires, that choice can come at the end of a process that reflects a binocular understanding of persons—an understanding that allows that persons are, and should be seen as, objects and subjects.

In chapter 3, "Creativity and Gratitude," I explore how a more binocular approach also aspires to oscillate between the "stances" that enthusiasts and critics adopt when they argue for or against the enhancement of human traits and capacities. In particular, I explore the deep and only apparently mutually exclusive insights that both sides bring to bear when they talk about the nature of human beings. Enthusiasts tend to emphasize that we are by nature creators and that we are true to our selves when we use technology to transform our selves. Critics, on the other hand, emphasize that we are by nature creatures and that by eschewing technological self-transformation, by affirming the way we were thrown into the world, we are true to our selves. Though one side emphasizes that we are creators, and the other that we are creatures, I will suggest that both sides share the moral ideal of authenticity and that we need both sides' insights if we're going to think deeply about the meaning of enhancement.

In chapter 4, "Technology as Value-Free and as Value-Laden," I describe the different lenses through which enthusiasts about and critics of technological intervention see what technology is. Specifically, I suggest that, whereas enthusiasts tend to see technology as a morally neutral or value-free tool, which we can put to whatever purposes we see fit, critics tend to see it as a value-laden frame, which shapes our purposes. Further, I call attention to how their different ways of seeing what technology *is* are entangled with their different ways of seeing what we *should* do with it. Once again, I emphasize the value of the insights on both sides, however partial they inevitably are.

In the next chapter, "Nobody's against True Enhancement," I gesture toward the sort of more binocular thinking about enhancement that we can engage in once we've gotten over taking a stand for or against it. Specifically, I will suggest that thinking in a more binocular way about the examples of love and memory can help us notice a simple but fundamental idea: no one is for an intervention that would separate us from the way we really are and the way the world really is—and no one should be against an intervention that would facilitate our ability to be in the world as we are and as it is. Moreover, I will emphasize an insight that the philosopher John Harris, a staunch and sometimes strident enthusiast about emerging technologies, makes in his book *Enhancing*

Evolution: The Ethical Case for Making Better People. I suggest that, if we should reject a technological intervention, it won't be on the grounds that the intervention is an enhancement, but on the grounds that it is not a "true" enhancement—on the grounds that it does not promote anyone's flourishing.

Chapter 6, "Comprehending Persons as Subjects and as Objects," is a bridge from the first five chapters of the book, which are concerned primarily with a binocular approach to thinking, to the last full chapter of the book, which is concerned primarily with a binocular approach to acting. In chapter 6 I turn to an approach to understanding persons, which elaborates the fundamental pair of lenses I introduced in chapter 2 ("Embracing Binocularity"): through one lens we see persons as free subjects and through the other as determined objects. Specifically, I explore how excitement regarding neuroscience (and allied sciences) can tempt us to lapse into a bad sort of "monocularity," where we see persons only as objects, and I suggest that we should, instead, get better at noticing and accepting the need for oscillating between the lenses.

In chapter 7, "Respecting Persons as Subjects and as Objects," I turn to that subset of technologically shaping selves debates concerned with using surgery to normalize the appearance of children with atypical bodies, from children with cleft lips and atypical genitalia to children with short limbs. I will say how a binocular approach to persons—seeing them as objects and as subjects— can inform a binocular approach to the process with which we make decisions in the clinic. Specifically I suggest that a binocular approach to persons can help us conceive the process of truly informed consent in terms of two stages. In the first, we recognize the way in which persons are objects, and we show them respect by challenging them to notice the forces that bear down on them and that shape their preference to refuse or request technological intervention. In the second stage (with rare exceptions), we recognize the way in which persons are subjects, and we show them respect by deferring to their truly informed decisions.

In the final part of the book, "Closing Thoughts," in addition to summarizing what a more binocular habit of thinking and acting would look like, I acknowledge that we may already be at the beginning of what I will call a "second wave" of the debates about technologically shaping our selves: one in which we are better than we were in the first wave at oscillating between the insights of those for whom criticism of technological intervention is congenial and the insights of those for whom enthusiasm is congenial. To the extent that a second wave has already begun, this book describes a problem of the past. However, to the extent that settling down and taking a rest with just one lens remains a permanent temptation, this book wrestles with a permanent problem.

Indeed, what interests me most, even more than the particulars of the debates about technologically shaping our selves, is the omnipresent problem of lapsing into using just one lens: seeing only from the vantage point that we find most congenial. As long as we are stuck with languages that perpetually produce binary distinctions—and as long as we are stuck with the desires to justify ourselves, to win arguments, and to conserve the amount of intellectual energy we expend in reaching our ethical conclusions—the temptation to think with only one lens will never disappear completely or for long.

It would be supremely ironic to imagine that binocularity is some sort of grand, meta-lens through which we can once and for all see what's at stake in the debates about technologically shaping our selves or in any other debates. Binocularity is neither more nor less than a metaphor, and it is imperfect in ways that I will rehearse in my concluding chapter. There I again emphasize that I don't offer binocularity as a cure or solution, but as the name for a habit of thinking that I have found helps me understand in more depth than the approach I adopted when I first began to engage in the debates about technologically shaping our selves. It is a habit of remembering that my insights are partial, both in the sense that they are always incomplete and in the sense that they reflect a stance toward the world that feels congenial to me. My hope is that in acknowledging and describing the partiality of my insights, I might make you more attuned to the partiality of yours. I would be elated if the habit of thinking I'm describing would be useful to all sorts of people engaged in all sorts of debates, but I will be quite satisfied if it is useful to people who are new to the debates about technologically shaping our selves.

Chapter 1

Seeing from Somewhere
in Particular

Perhaps like most fields of human inquiry, bioethics is not just one thing and did not spring up in one pristine place or at one magical moment. Nonetheless, it's fair to say that what today we call the field of bioethics, with all the trappings of an academic field, including university degrees, fellowships, professional organizations, and government-funded grants, emerged in the United States in the late 1960s and early '70s.[1]

Into that new field flowed multiple and in some cases ancient streams. At least since the 4th century B.C.E., when Hippocrates wrote about the nature of disease and the obligations of physicians to patients, some form of medical ethics has been around. The more recent stream of research ethics, which reached international consciousness with news of how Nazi doctors used human beings in their experiments, was around in inchoate form at least since the beginning of the 20th century, when the great physician William Osler suggested that there is a "sacred cord which binds physician and patient" and that it would "snap" if physicians performed experiments that did not directly benefit patients.[2]

By the late 1960s and early '70s, many of the most pressing questions in those two bioethical streams could ultimately be answered with an appeal to the hugely important, widely shared, and increasingly noncontroversial value of autonomy (or one of its cognates, such as liberty or freedom). The answer was to let individuals decide for themselves. In its commitment to promoting the research subject's or patient's right to decide for herself (whether to participate in a trial or whether to receive treatment), bioethics was akin to other social movements of the day, including those that advanced the rights of women, people of color, sexual minorities, and people with disabilities. All of those movements sought to secure the full right to self-determination for people who formerly had been denied it.[3]

Such a "procedural" answer to practical ethical questions, one that recommends how a decision-making process should go rather than what the outcome should be, is thoroughly and deeply ethical. It is an answer that I will, after careful explication, endorse at the end of this book—and that, as I will acknowledge, is not nearly as bold or as exciting as I would wish. It is an approach grounded in an appeal to the goodness of allowing persons to choose their own ways for themselves, with the understanding that they, better than anyone else, can know what will promote their own flourishing. It is grounded in the same substantive ethical commitment that found unparalleled expression in John Stuart Mill's *On Liberty*.

So long as we notice the way in which the approach to answering those questions is procedural, it can make sense to speak of bioethical "expertise."[4] Clinical bioethicists, for example, can have expertise in facilitating conversations among patients, nurses, physicians, and others who can help patients answer for themselves the practical question, What should I do? The bioethicist's expertise is in helping the patient explore what the various options mean for her, in helping her determine whether a given intervention will promote her flourishing as she understands it. Research bioethicists can have expertise regarding not only how to craft informed consent forms and the increasingly complex regulations that govern such research, but also the histories of the fundamental values involved in competing proposals for new strategies to regulate such research. And bioethicists who specialize in thinking about the just distribution of scarce health care resources can have expertise regarding the mechanisms that deliver those resources and also the histories of the fundamental values involved in competing proposals for distributing them. When we speak of expertise in such contexts, however, the expertise refers to knowing which questions to ask and which procedures will promote their asking. It doesn't refer to the answers to the "meaning questions" that are always at play.

MEANING QUESTIONS

As soon as we begin asking not only what we have a right to do but also what we ought to do, we find ourselves asking meaning questions. What we think we ought to do depends, in significant measure, on what we think it means to be human. It depends on what sorts of beings we think we are—on our tentative answers to questions like, What does working well, or flourishing, look like in organisms like us? What makes us truly happy? What, if any, are the proper roles of suffering and death in our lives? What is the proper relationship between parents and children? And, among myriad others, What is our proper stance toward our selves and the rest of the world?

Insofar as using technology to shape the world and thus ultimately our selves has always been a crucial feature of being human, reflecting on the difference between the proper and improper uses of technology has been an ancient preoccupation. That is, asking questions about the proper uses of technology has long been a way of asking questions about the meaning of being human. These are questions that the authors of Genesis were grappling with when they imagined human beings who were creative enough to build a tower into the heavens. They are the questions that the authors of the myth of Icarus grappled with when they imagined a human being so inventive as to be able to fly near the sun. And they are the questions that Plato was reflecting on when, in the *Phaedrus*, he worried that the technology of writing corrupted human beings, by effectively banishing their older, purer method of transmitting stories from memory.

So questions, and worries, about the meaning of technology, and about the difference between the proper and improper uses of it, are nothing new. But those questions gained urgency in the late 1960s and early '70s, when ever more technologies that promised to transform our selves were emerging: from drugs and surgeries aimed at what was called "mind control" to reproductive and genetic technologies that promised to let parents choose their children's traits. Today, as at the time of the birth of bioethics as a field, meaning questions are nowhere more palpable than in the discussion of how we should use new technologies to shape our children and ourselves.

As the philosophically minded psychoanalyst and Hastings Center cofounder Willard Gaylin would say, the questions we ask today about the meaning of technologically shaping our selves are old wine in new bottles: ancient questions in the context of the newest advances in science, medicine, and technology. One could fairly say, though, that there's a way in which the field of bioethics "saved the life of" those questions,[5] and a way in which Gaylin and Callahan's founding of The Hastings Center was an act of rebellion. By calling attention to the ancient questions raised by advances in science, medicine, and technology, they rejected the Anglo-American philosophical orthodoxy of the day, which suggested that grownups should stick with questions that at least appeared to admit of crisp answers,[6] questions like, Which conditions must an utterance meet to warrant being called true? Callahan and Gaylin were suggesting, instead, that grownups should tolerate the frustration that goes with asking the questions that Milan Kundera once said "even a child can ask."[7] The ones that don't admit of crisp or final answers are, Kundera averred, "the only truly serious questions."[8]

What I'm getting at is this: at our best, we in bioethics honor the impossibility of final answers to meaning questions *and* we honor the necessity of answering practical ethical questions. At our worst, we pretend to possess expert answers to those enduring meaning questions: we indulge the wizard fantasy that I mentioned in the introduction—either our own fantasy that we are wizards, or the fantasy of others that bioethical wizards exist.

COMING TO MEANING QUESTIONS FROM SOMEWHERE IN PARTICULAR

I suggest that, despite the absence of final answers to meaning questions, we need to keep the conversation about them going. I understand how obvious that suggestion might sound at first, but unfortunately it is not, not when ever more of us imagine that the only questions worth asking admit of crisp answers: ones that will protect people from physical harm, or improve their health, or grow the economy. Not only can it be hard to justify asking meaning questions in a world teeming with the other, harder-nosed sort, but asking such questions can be difficult. Engaging in conversation where real speaking and listening happens between people whose stances toward the world are really different is harder and rarer than it sounds. To begin with, it requires getting better at acknowledging that each of us comes to these questions from somewhere in particular.

When I say that each of us comes to the technologically shaping selves debates from somewhere in particular, partly I mean to emphasize that each of us comes to the debates from a particular stance toward the world.[i] None of us reasoned our way to the stance that feels right to us. Were we to more fully recognize that, we might be less prone to speak as if we came from reason alone and our interlocutors from feeling (or intuition or emotion).

When I say that each of us comes to these debates from somewhere in particular, I also mean that each of us comes to any bioethical question from our own life experience. "Oh, really?" you might be asking. "And is there salt in the sea?" As painfully obvious as that point is, when we make bioethical (and other) sorts of arguments, we often forget it. That forgetfulness puts us at significantly increased risk of exaggerating the value of our reasons and conclusions and at equally great risk of missing the value of others' reasons and conclusions.

Because I hate the endless personal strip teasing that we seem to demand of each other today, I will keep mine to a minimum. But I can't simply skip it. I, too, come to the questions concerning technologically shaping selves from somewhere in particular. And I am committed to remembering Kay Redfield Jamison's true and

---

i For a rich and sympathetic account of the role of philosophical "stances" in the articulation of ethical conclusions, which can be traced at least back to David Hume, see Gregory Kaebnick's *Humans in Nature: The World as We Find It and the World as We Create It* (New York: Oxford University Press, 2014). See, too, Jonathan Haidt's *The Righteous Mind: Why Good People Are Divided by Politics and Religion* (New York: Pantheon, 2012).

demanding words: "One is what one is, and the dishonesty of hiding behind a degree, or a title, or any manner and collection of words is still exactly that: dishonesty."[9]

Growing up I thought of myself as melancholic, and I accepted that that was just who I was. Moreover, I could pretty easily weave my ongoing unhappiness into a story about the history of my family.

On May 1, 1942, when my father was 13, his mother helped him escape from an internment camp in the south of France, where they were both detained. His mother understood where the internees were headed, although not in the detail we do now. On August 14, 1942, my father's mother, Rosa Prusinowski, was put on a train at the Le Bourget-Drancy station, in a suburb of Paris, headed for Auschwitz. My father would never again see a single member of his large, extended family. In spite of the fundamental love and material comforts of my youth, our family lived against the horizon of the Shoah.

When I was young, my mother, a poet, was drawn to the likes of Sylvia Plath and Anne Sexton. Sadness seemed eminently reasonable and actually admirable. I would look around at my schoolmates and neighbors and ask myself, What's wrong with those people who aren't unhappy? Don't they know anything about world history? Don't they see the cruelty and suffering all around us? Don't they understand anything about human nature? I took my unhappiness to be a sign of the depth of my character and understanding.

But I reached a point where, regardless of the depth of character that my unhappiness did or didn't signal, I reluctantly accepted that I needed help. I spent four or five years in college and graduate school undergoing a low-cost psychoanalysis with an analyst in training. The young doctor was as thoughtful and sensitive as

I could have wished, and reflecting on my life, three or four days a week, was interesting, but it didn't put a dent in my unhappiness.

After the sometimes harrowing nine-year journey to receiving my PhD, I, as I mentioned earlier, had a string of one- and two-year teaching posts. During one of them, in North Carolina, I spent a couple more years doing talk therapy with a wonderful social worker, which almost always made me feel better temporarily but didn't relieve my unhappiness. During my next post, I visited the physician responsible for the care of the students and faculty at the college in Indiana where I taught. He became alarmed at my symptoms: unrelenting insomnia, severe irritability, deep sense of worthlessness, and so on. When he recommended Prozac, I was taken aback. Surely prescription drugs are only for people who are really sick, and I was just really unhappy. I'm not sure if it was something about his no-nonsense Midwestern manner, or my realization that if I didn't do something I might never leave that lovely, but to me wholly alien, town, but I decided to try it.

The drug made me feel better. After a couple of decades of feeling unhappy, feeling okay was strange, but welcome. Unfortunately, the dose I was prescribed also produced intolerable side effects, so I quit after about six months. That, however, was long enough to land a job at The Hastings Center, meet my soon-to-be wife, and start a new life in New York. After that truncated use of the drug, I didn't give it much more thought.

THE ENHANCEMENT QUESTION

In 1993, however, a year after I arrived at The Hastings Center, Peter Kramer published *Listening to Prozac.* Kramer explicitly stated that his book was not about treating depression, but about making people, as he famously put it, "feel better than well."[10] Of course, partly, my own experience of Prozac as a treatment explains my interest in Kramer's book. At least as much, though, the book grabbed my attention because the idea of using a medical technology to "enhance" our selves ran absolutely counter to one of my deepest ethical intuitions: that there is something good about accepting and affirming the way we are thrown into the world.

The highly respected bioethicist LeRoy Walters evoked the same intuition in me when, right around the same time that Kramer's book was published, he gave a talk at The Hastings Center. In his inimitably clear, thoughtful, and gentle way, Walters suggested that it might become possible and ethically desirable to use genetic technology to make human beings less aggressive and more kind.[11] When I heard that suggestion, I became nearly apoplectic. Isn't aggression a difficult but essential part of a fully human life? If we sought to remove such aggression, mightn't we inadvertently reduce the likelihood that we would achieve great things? Hadn't he read Homer, for God's sake? Could Achilles have achieved greatness without his anger?

After reading Kramer and listening to Walters, I decided to put together a grant application to do a project on what I then called "enhancement technologies." It was my first major grant application, and it gave me a chance to engage with a question I felt passionately about. Moreover, I hoped it would give me a chance to do what I had always dreamed of: to stand up and say, Absolutely No! I would be different from those cowardly monsters of the 1930s and '40s: I would say No to my own time's form of dehumanization.

So, motivated at least in part by a deep intuition about the wrongness of enhancement and by a strong desire to stand up and say No, I promised our funder that the working group of philosophers, health policy experts, sociologists, and others that I put together would not only investigate the broad, fundamental philosophical questions about the meaning of using new technologies to enhance human traits and capacities, but also articulate guidelines for (unspecified) policy makers, which would distinguish between acceptable and unacceptable uses of new medical technologies. I assumed that, by carefully articulating the difference between treatment and enhancement, we could then move on to endorse treatments and censure enhancements.

TREATMENT VS. ENHANCEMENT

The project included lengthy debates about whether the treatment-enhancement distinction was conceptually coherent.[12] Those who were critical of the prospect of enhancement tended to argue for the coherence of the distinction. To do that, we had to in one way or another appeal to nature, specifically, to one or another variation on the idea that, whereas treatment restores normal or species-typical human functioning, enhancement does more than that. Those who were enthusiastic about enhancement, on the other hand, argued that the distinction was too fuzzy to be useful. Given that human traits (from blood pressure to stress tolerance) are distributed continuously in a population, they argued, it just isn't possible to discern bright lines between typical and atypical functioning.

The charge of fuzziness is not necessarily fatal to all efforts to use the treatment-enhancement distinction. As the old saw would have it, just because it's hard to say at dawn whether it's night or day doesn't mean we can't distinguish the two. Nor is it fatal to the distinction to observe, as some disability theorists did,[13] that the distinction smuggles in pernicious assumptions about the goodness of normality or species typicality. We could, after all, be vigilant about criticizing such assumptions. Indeed, it might be that, if we were to attempt to create a just health care system, we would have to distinguish between services we could afford and ones we couldn't, and that a highly imperfect, potentially dangerous distinction like the one between treatment and enhancement would be one of many tools to help figure out what should and shouldn't go into a basic package of medical care.

In addition to assuming that the treatment-enhancement distinction was coherent, however, my grant application made another assumption that was, if anything, more problematic. This assumption had to do with the goals of medicine:[14] both with what those goals are and with the putative ethical implications of identifying them. Specifically, when I initiated the enhancement project, I tacitly hoped that, once we explicated the difference between the medical goal of treatment and the nonmedical goal of enhancement, and once we established that the technologies at issue (surgery, pharmacology, genetics) were medical technologies, we would have established that enhancement was beyond the ethical pale, insofar as it was inconsistent with the goals of medicine. If, for example, a new drug could do more than treat someone's unhappiness, making her happier than she "normally" or "naturally" would be, it would be beyond the ethical pale.

The philosopher James Lindemann Nelson, however, invited members of the project working group to see the flaw in that line of reasoning. He said, Okay, let's assume, for the sake of argument, that we can specify what the proper goals of medicine are. We can then agree that *doctors* should not offer interventions that are inconsistent with those goals. But, Nelson suggested, let's imagine another human activity called "schmedicine," which has its own goals and which is practiced by "schmoctors." It wouldn't make sense to criticize a schmoctor on the grounds that she wasn't pursuing the goals of medicine; those aren't her goals. The goals-of-medicine argument wouldn't have ethical force for the schmoctor.

I'm glad that in my final project report[15] I didn't suggest that the treatment-enhancement distinction could alone provide guidance even for physicians or medical insurance companies, much less for "schmoctors." I only suggested that it might be one tool among many for saying something about what should go into a basic package of medical care. True to my fundamental intuition—my fundamental feeling—about the goodness of learning to let things be and thus the potential badness of enhancement, however, I did identify concerns that "our society" ought to have about such interventions, whether they were offered by a doctor or a schmoctor. I described the kinds of problems that might be exacerbated if schmoctors or anyone else started peddling new technologies to achieve enhancement: for example, such technologies might exacerbate the gap between the haves and have-nots, or might facilitate people becoming complicit with ethically suspect norms, or might aid people in becoming untrue to themselves or inauthentic.

You may have noticed that in the preceding paragraph, I referred to my "fundamental *intuition*" regarding the goodness of learning to let things be, and I also suggested its relation to a "fundamental *feeling*" about the goodness of learning to let things be. Admittedly, I don't have a worked-out view of the precise relation between intuition and feeling, but I will use those two terms, and emotion as well, to call attention to an element in my own ethical judgments and in the ethical judgments of others, which is more than reason alone.[ii]

I should emphasize that I am absolutely *not* suggesting that intuition or feeling or emotion can serve as any sort of ethical anchor, guide, or special source of wisdom.[16] I am eager, though, to recognize the presence of that element in all ethical judgments— even in the ethical judgments of people who sometimes sound as if they believe that they are especially good at speaking "impartially," from reason alone.[17] My point is not that "partiality" is good, nor is it that we should defer to feeling. My point is that, when we debate the sorts of meaning questions at issue in this book, it is inevitable that our insights will be "partial"—both in the sense that they will not be complete and in the sense that we have a special affection for them. They feel right to us. Failing to recognize the role of feeling or intuition in reaching our ethical conclusions is as dangerous as failing to aspire to give reasons for our conclusions.

DIFFERENT INTUITIONS

One place in which to see intuition play out in the conclusions of critics and enthusiasts about enhancement is in the debates about preimplantation genetic diagnosis (PGD), the procedure whereby fertility specialists ascertain the genetic profile of an embryo before transferring it to a woman's uterus. On the one side, critics have the intuition that

ii For an overview of current debates among moral psychologists regarding the relationship between what I have here called "reason" and "emotion," see Jonathan Haidt and Selin Kesebir, "Morality," in Susan Fiske, Daniel Gilbert, and Gardner Linkzey, eds. *Handbook of Social Psychology, 5th Edition* (Hoboken, N.J.: Wiley, 2010), 797–832; and Jonathan Haidt, "The New Synthesis in Moral Psychology," *Science* 316, no. 5827 (2007): 998–1001.

we should affirm what the pioneering disability rights activist Harriet McBryde Johnson called "the muck and mess" of life.[18] They have the intuition that there is goodness in affirming a wide variety of forms of being human, including the messy form that McBryde took, with her atrophied muscles and thus inability to walk or bathe or eat without assistance. They argue that using PGD to "weed out" embryos destined for lives like McBryde's is a mistake.[19] On the other side, enthusiasts have the intuition that we should clean up the muck and mess. They have the intuition that it is bad to knowingly bring children with disabilities into the world, and they argue that there is a moral obligation to bring into the world "the best possible baby."[20]

As philosophically minded PGD enthusiasts have long recognized, however, that intuition creates a knotty logical problem:[21] it is maddeningly difficult to give unassailable reasons for why it is bad to bring a child with a disability into the world. After all, if parents choose to bring into existence an embryo (or fetus) that has a disabling trait, they have not harmed *that* child. No matter how difficult life with the disabling trait might be, life with disability is almost always preferable to the alternative of nonexistence.

There is now a large, not-always-fun-to-read literature, which seeks to untie that knot, to give reasons to support the enthusiasts' intuition that it is bad to knowingly bring a child with a disability into the world, even though that child couldn't otherwise exist.[22] The most common approach is utilitarian, and it essentially suggests that we shift our frame of reference. On such an approach, we should stop thinking in terms of how a particular decision would affect a particular person (in this case, the person who would develop from whichever embryo were chosen in the context of PGD), and we should start thinking in terms of how this decision would affect the aggregate welfare or happiness of society. Once we shift to such an approach, we will see that it's unethical to bring a person with a disability into the world because, other things being equal, more disability means less total welfare.

While the utilitarian philosopher Peter Singer would deny that his view about the badness of disability is in any damning sense based on an intuition, he does, to his credit, acknowledge that intuitions are always at work in ethics. He grants that "even a radical ethical theory like utilitarianism must rest on a fundamental intuition about what is good."[23] Singer suggests, however, that we have to distinguish between types of intuition. Specifically, he urges us to distinguish between intuitions that are rooted in our evolutionary past and ones that he suggests are rooted in reason. The fact that you feel more love for your children than you do for your cousin's children, whom you love more than children who are not genetically related to you, has long evolutionary roots. But, Singer observes, that sort of intuition is different in kind from and inferior to, say, the intuition that "the good of any one individual is of no more importance, from the point of view... of the Universe, than the good of any other."[24]

That beautiful intuition about the equal moral value of all persons, which is at the very heart of Singer's work, can also, of course, be found in the world's great religions. As from the point of view of the Universe, from the point of view of God, the good of any one individual is no more important than the good of any other. But when disability rights activists and their fellow travelers hear Singer and his fellow enthusiasts speak, they sometimes fear they hear echoes of another intuition that can also be found in the world's great religions: the intuition that we are destined for another better, purer, cleaner place. In the utilitarian's call to stop knowingly bringing children with disabilities into the world, there is a trace of the ancient intuition that we need to clean up the human "muck and mess."

REASONS AND INTUITIONS

Invariably, as soon as anyone suggests that intuition, feeling, or emotion plays a role in constituting ethical positions, one of her interlocutors will be quick to ask, Are you suggesting that reason plays no role? Are you suggesting that ethical positions are no more than rationalizations of gut reactions? Do you think that the badness of slavery is a matter of "intuition"? What about Nazism? What about child trafficking and homophobia?

I am not suggesting any of that. I am saying, however, that if we are to get better at pursuing meaning questions together, we need to get better at really noticing the particularity of our starting places—including the particularity of our intuitions, feelings, and emotions—not to mention our material interests (which is a gigantically important topic for someone else's book). Saying such a thing is not the same as taking a stand for feeling or against reason. It is not to suggest that ethical conclusions are always *only* rationalizations of feelings or intuitions. Nor is it to say that all intuitions or feelings deserve equal respect. But it is to insist that, as a matter of fact, reasons and intuitions (or feelings or emotions) play a role in reaching ethical conclusions, both good and bad ones.[25]

Whereas Singer appeals to evolutionary theory to distinguish between intuitions or feelings rooted in our natural history and ones rooted in reason, Martha Nussbaum appeals to psychoanalytic theory to distinguish between, on the one hand, feelings that are projections onto others of what we find disgusting and fearful in ourselves (from our feces to our mortality) and, on the other, feelings that are rooted in our sense of justice. As Nussbaum observes, it is one thing to *feel disgust* toward people who have homosexual sex (or who have disabilities) and quite another to *feel indignation* at harms done to people who have homosexual sex (or have disabilities).[26] Nussbaum wants us to get over our feelings of disgust toward others, which she takes to be rooted in our fear and denial of our own animality and mortality. She wants us to overcome what she says is our longing "to get away from messy, sticky humanity."[27]

It seems to me that Singer and Nussbaum are exactly right to attempt to distinguish between, as it were, more and less constructive forms of intuition or feeling, and my guess is that Nussbaum's approach may ultimately bear more fruit. For now, though, I am only suggesting that more and less constructive forms of intuition or feeling are at work on both sides of the debates about technologically shaping our selves and that those debates would advance more productively if we could give up the notion that any of us ever proceeds from reason alone. There is nothing to be lost and much to be gained by owning up to the entanglement of the reasons and feelings that give rise to our ethical conclusions.

ONE SORT OF ANXIOLYTIC

After the publication of the final report and volume of essays[28] from my "enhancement" project, I started to be invited to give talks about the ethics of enhancement. When lecture organizers invite a bioethicist to speak, they're usually looking for a wizard with a PowerPoint—someone who can, in 45 minutes, make a case and take a stand. They want to be told if a given practice, whether it's paid organ donation, research on embryos, or enhancement, is right or wrong. (Funders of bioethics research also often want the same thing.) Because my own intuition about enhancement was so negative, initially it was easy to deliver what my hosts expected: an argument *against*.

The basic bioethical dance is pretty simple. The first step, in a show of appearing open to the insights on the other side, is to present one's opponent's arguments. The second step is to try to demolish them. In my case, this meant setting up, in preparation for taking down, the arguments *for* enhancement. The net result would, of course, be that my arguments against enhancement would prevail.

An upside of taking a stand and just saying No!—*or* Yes!—is that one gets to revel in the sentiment of one's own moral courage. A downside is that taking such a stand on a truly complex question can be anxiety producing and energy consuming. After all, it takes considerable energy to try to demolish a view, if, as in most cases, it contains some insight. And it takes equally much energy to deflect one's opponent's criticism, if, as in most cases, it contains some insight.

At least for me, it was anxiety producing to speak publicly as if I believed that my criticism of enhancement was right, full stop, and my opponent's enthusiasm was wrong, full stop. Moreover, going through the choreographed moves—failing to truly acknowledge the defects in my view and the insights in the other—was wholly inconsistent with the Socratic approach to learning I came to love as a student.

If one spends less energy denying the insight on the other side and exaggerating the insight on one's own, one has more energy to spend on trying to understand the meaning of whatever is at hand. Sustaining the tension between insights might itself create a sort of anxiety, but it is of a more fruitful sort than the one associated with trying to win the point. Of course, not all questions call for the sort of understanding I'm after. As I just indicated, I wouldn't suggest that we need a deeper understanding of the question concerning the meaning of slavery. I want to insist, however, that the meaning of "enhancement"—or, as I will put it later, "true improvement"—is a different sort of beast and demands a different sort of approach.

Chapter 2

Embracing Binocularity

In the previous chapter, I suggested that the meaning questions that arise in the debates about enhancement don't admit of crisp or final answers and that, nonetheless, thinking about those questions is an ineliminable part of deciding how we should live. In this chapter, I want to say more about what I will refer to as a "binocular" habit of thinking about those questions. I take this habit of thinking to be more fruitful than the one I adopted when I began engaging in the debates about enhancement, and to be useful for thinking about technologically shaping our selves more broadly. Before I say more about this approach, however, I should say a bit more about what I mean by "technologically shaping our selves."

When I say that we are shaping our *selves* with technology, I mean to emphasize that whether someone uses a scalpel to shape her body or a drug to shape her brain, she does so to shape her experience—to alter what it is like for her to be her. A drug like Prozac, for example, can, by changing someone's brain chemistry, change what it feels like to be in the world, which can affect how one is treated by others, which, in turn, can further shape one's experience of what it is like to be her. Surgeries to lengthen the limbs of a child with dwarfism aim to improve her ability to navigate a social world built for people of typical height, but they also can aim to improve how she is experienced by others and thereby improve her experience of her self. Whether the technological intervention affects someone's experience by changing her brain or by changing her body, the aim is to shape her self.

Because I want to remain as close as possible to the world as we know it, when I refer to *technologically* shaping our selves, I have been invoking and will continue to invoke examples of pharmacological and surgical technologies. So I will not talk much about using, for example, genetic technologies or nanotechnologies to shape our selves.[1] I should point out, however, that the insights that enthusiasts and critics bring to bear in the context of discussing more futuristic technologies are hard if not impossible to distinguish from the insights they bring to bear in the context of any other technology that promises to shape our selves. The technologies change, but the ethical insights and arguments on both sides remain largely, if not entirely, the same.

The insights and arguments for and against technological self-shaping can, to a surprising extent, also remain largely the same even as the specific purpose or aim of the technological shaping changes. As I have already mentioned, one of the classic aims discussed in these debates is to make someone "better than normal," as in the case of a pill that could enhance the mood of a healthy person.[2] Technological interventions can also aim to make someone "more normal," as in the case of a surgery to repair a cleft lip.[3] Sometimes the technology at issue aims to make someone "less normal," as with a surgery to remove the healthy limb of someone who says she can't otherwise feel whole.[4] Sometimes it aims to make someone "*better than* just better than normal," as in an imagined genetic technology of the future that would allow us to achieve what the philosopher Nicholas Agar calls radical enhancement: interventions that give us, for example, cognitive powers that exceed Einstein's or musical powers that exceed

Mozart's.[5] And sometimes the technology at issue aims to mock the idea of normal, as in the case of someone who deploys implants, piercings, and tattoos across every inch of her epidermis.[6] Again, just as the insights and arguments hardly change from technology to technology, they hardly change from aim to aim.

BINOCULARITY

While the term *binocularity* isn't used much in plain English, it is an apt name for the habit of thinking that I am suggesting can help us engage the meaning questions that arise in debates like the ones concerning technologically shaping our selves. This habit requires constantly remembering that, if we want deeper understanding—and ultimately better action—we need to aspire to think with at least two "lenses" at once. Much as our brains achieve visual depth perception by integrating the slightly different information that our two eyes give us, we can achieve depth of understanding by integrating the greatly different insights that at least two conceptual lenses give us.

Please notice that, in qualifying the phrase "two conceptual lenses" with the phrase "at least," I intend to make a couple of points. First, two lenses may not be enough to enable us to perfectly comprehend even just one facet of a given issue. Just because our languages so constantly produce binary oppositions—just because so many conceptual lenses come in pairs—shouldn't make us imagine that any given pair is enough. Maybe, to take an example I'll explore in a moment, it isn't enough to comprehend persons only as subjects and as objects. Maybe perfect comprehension would require using a third or thirtieth lens as well.

The second point I'm getting at with the phrase "at least" is that, even if one pair of lenses can sometimes be enough to understand one facet of a given ethical issue, one pair of lenses surely won't be enough to understand the whole issue. If, for example, the issue we're grappling with is whether someone should use a technology to shape her self, it would hardly suffice to consider that the person who is contemplating the intervention is a subject and is an object! As we will see, we need to consider many other facets of the issue, including, just to start, what we take human nature to be, what we think technology is, what nature is, what disability is, what human flourishing is, and so forth. Perhaps someone built for perfect comprehension would use an infinite number of lenses, from an infinite number of distances, and at an infinite number of angles. In this book, however, my aspiration is quite a bit more modest. It is to resist the temptation to use just one lens, at one distance, from one angle—and to achieve the deeper sort of comprehension that can come with using at least two lenses. As we will see, just using two lenses at once is harder than it sounds.

I first encountered the metaphor of binocularity in Jonathan Glover's essay "Towards Humanism in Psychiatry," where he writes:

> When we see the physical world in depth, we make use of having two eyes. The brain decodes the slightly discrepant pictures from the two eyes to get information about the relative distance of things. Knowledge of depth is extracted from the incompatibilities. This can be a metaphor for aspects of psychiatry. It is a field in which there are truths that at first can seem incompatible. We create ourselves, to some extent; yet

what we are like is also quite severely constrained by factors outside our control.[7]

Glover introduces the metaphor in his description of what we need to do if we are to comprehend persons who are diagnosed with psychiatric disorders. For such comprehension, he says, we need to integrate two different "pictures" of ourselves; in one "we create ourselves, to some extent," and in the other we are "quite severely constrained by factors outside our control." In my formulation, to comprehend persons with psychiatric disorders we need to see them with two conceptual lenses; we need to see them as subjects who are free to create themselves and as objects whose actions are determined by factors outside their control.

Of course it is not only persons with psychiatric disorders who need to be seen with two lenses if they are to be comprehended in depth. The same holds for all persons. In Glover's later book, *Choosing Children*, where he discusses healthy parents contemplating choices regarding the characteristics of their future children, he makes that same point in different language: he suggests we need to understand persons both "from the inside" and, as it were, "from the outside."[8]

From the inside, or first-person, perspective, persons have subjective experience. There is something *that it is like*[9] to have the experience of choosing freely, just as there is something that it is like to have the experience of shame, pride, love, hate, delight, despair, hope, fear, envy, admiration, and all the rest. Though we can't ever have certain knowledge of what it is like for someone else to be herself, we can come to understand much about what her experience is like, what it means to her, by asking her. We can also come to understand much about what it is like, in general, to have such experiences, by turning to painters, novelists, playwrights, poets, anthropologists, historians, and philosophers.

Glover observes that we also need to consider a person through the object lens. We need to comprehend the forces and mechanisms that explain how her experience emerges out of matter. We need to comprehend the forces and mechanisms that constitute her, that converge in the site that she is. Here we can draw on the third-person perspective of the sciences. (The distinction between a third-person perspective that is concerned with explanation and a first-person perspective that is concerned with understanding has a long history; one of the first most notable articulators of that distinction is the 19th-century German philosopher Wilhelm Dilthey.[10])

I should reiterate that the two lenses do not let us see two different entities in the sense of letting us see two different substances. The metaphor of binocularity does not entail any sort of dualism, according to which persons are a composite of one substance that has extension (the body) and a second that does not (the mind).[i] Nor does the metaphor of binocularity allow for any grand reduction, according to which mind is really body (as the materialist would have it) or according to which body is really mind (as the idealist would have it).[11] I take Glover to be suggesting that we need both lenses equally if we are to comprehend persons in depth.

---

i Though the metaphor of binocularity most certainly does not entail any sort of *substance* dualism, it might be said to entail a sort of *semantic* dualism, understood as a view that recognizes the need for at least two languages to talk about the one phenomenon that is the person (Jean-Pierre Changeux and Paul Ricoeur, *What Makes Us Think? A Neuroscientist and a Philosopher Argue about Ethics, Human Nature, and the Brain* [Princeton, N.J.: Princeton University Press: 2000]). For a Wittgensteinian twist on the same idea, see Gregory E. Kaebnick, "Behavioral Genetics and Moral Responsibility," in *Wrestling with Behavioral Genetics: Science, Ethics, and Public Conversation*, ed. Erik Parens, Audrey Chapman, and Nancy Press (Baltimore, Md.: Johns Hopkins University Press, 2005).

In my attempt to articulate a more binocular habit of thinking and, ultimately, acting, I use the metaphor of binocularity in the specific way that Glover does—urging us to remember that we are objects and subjects—and I use it in at least three additional ways. First, I urge us to notice the value of oscillating between the "stances" from which we come to the debates about technologically shaping our selves. Second, I urge us to notice the value of oscillating between the insights seen through the various pairs of conceptual lenses (including, but not limited to, the subject and object lenses) that we invoke when we argue for the conclusion that feels right from our "stance." Finally, I suggest the sense in which comprehending persons first as objects and then as subjects can help us conceive of and help facilitate a process of truly informed consent.

A MORE BINOCULAR HABIT OF THINKING
ABOUT OUR STANCES

If we were to adopt a more binocular habit of thinking, we would become better at recognizing that critics come to these debates from a stance—or cluster of insights and intuitions—that feels right to them, and enthusiasts come from a different stance that feels equally right to them. A more binocular approach requires recognizing the extent to which, while one stance will inevitably feel more congenial to us than will the other, the other isn't wholly uncongenial. It requires getting better at oscillating between the stances of the critics and enthusiasts. It means refusing for as long as possible to choose for or against technological intervention in general, and it means seeking to promote a conversation about the meaning of "true improvement" in a given context. As we will see in the next chapter, the critics of and enthusiasts regarding such attempts are both seeing and saying important things from their different stances, and a binocular approach gains depth of comprehension by benefiting from both. In particular, both sides share a commitment to facilitating persons' efforts to engage in activities in the world as they are and as the world is.

You may have just noticed, however, that in my call to get over the big binary choice between being for and against enhancement, I rather quickly, if tacitly, introduced a new binary. After all, the phrase "true improvement" entails a binary opposite, such as "fake (or false) improvement." You might wonder, that is, if I exhibit the illness I say we need to treat. And your diagnosis would be right. I do, and there is no cure. Using very different terms, the postmodernist philosopher Jacques Derrida broached this same fundamental riddle when he wrote:

> There is no sense in doing without the concepts of metaphysics in order to shake metaphysics. We have no language—no syntax and no lexicon—which is foreign to this history; *we can pronounce not a single destructive proposition which has not already had to slip into the form, the logic, and the implicit postulations of precisely what it seeks to contest* [emphasis added].[12]

I want to contest the system of binary oppositions that would have us choose between being for and against technologically achieved improvement of our selves, and in my contestation I end up invoking the binary opposition between true and fake improvement. From this I do not infer that I should try harder to get free of such binaries, but that I need to remember that there is no getting free of them. In lieu of a cure, we do our best to remember that we have the disease, and we try to reduce its worst flare-ups.

A MORE BINOCULAR HABIT OF THINKING
ABOUT BASIC CONCEPTS

I also use the metaphor of binocularity to describe a habit of think-ing about some of the "smaller" binary choices we make when we offer a defense of our big binary choice for or against technologi-cally shaping our selves. Here I have in mind choices regarding some of the basic concepts that are deployed in these debates—such as technology, nature, and disability. We can get much better at resisting, for longer, the temptation to speak as if, for example, technology is a value-free tool *or* a value-laden frame; as if nature is a mechanism that we can engineer *or* a fragile web that we should let be; or as if disability is a medical fact *or* a social construction. Our comprehension of any of those concepts will be deeper if we attempt to use at least two lenses at once.

And it is essential to notice that, in practice, we can't actually think with any two lenses at once, whether we're talking about the subject and object lenses or the lenses offered by the medical and social models of disability. To get this point, which is absolutely central to this book, it can help to recall the figure that was first introduced by gestalt psychologists and then made famous by Ludwig Wittgenstein in his *Philosophical Investigations*: the figure that can look like either a duck or a rabbit, depending on how you focus your attention.[13] I am suggesting that we can no more see ourselves, for example, as objects and as subjects at the same time than we can see that figure as a rabbit and as a duck at the same time.[ii] In practice, we can see ourselves as an object and then as a subject, but we can't do both at once.

---

ii Ellen K. Feder makes an analogous point about seeing gender and race in *Family Bonds: Genealogies of Race and Gender* (New York: Oxford University Press, 2007).

Because we aren't built for thinking in a perfectly binocular way, for actually using two lenses at once, we need to accept imperfect ways. I call the imperfect way at the center of this book "oscillating binocularity." In the absence of the capacity to think with two lenses at once, oscillating binocularity requires the discipline and energy to shuttle back and forth between the sorts of lenses I have already mentioned. And make no mistake: oscillating between lenses requires more intellectual energy than settling down and taking a rest with just one.

When I suggest in the title of this chapter that we should embrace binocularity, I mean to imply a contrast to our all-too-human tendency to flee it. It is true that, as I alluded to in the preceding chapter, fleeing binocularity requires energy. But embracing binocularity—aspiring to use two lenses at once— requires much more. In fact, my experience as a participant in the debates about technologically shaping our selves has sometimes made me wonder if we should consider the first law of thinking dynamics to be the Law of the Conservation of Mental Energy, according to which, when we think about ethical questions—and of course many other sorts of questions as well—we tend to use as little mental energy as is compatible with continuing to fancy ourselves intellectually respectable. Our natural tendency is to lapse into using just one lens, into what I will call "monocularity."

TWO SORTS OF MONOCULARITY

I just identified a respect in which perfectly binocular thinking is humanly impossible. I also need to acknowledge a respect in which it can become morally undesirable. To explain what I mean, it will help to explicate this book's two epigraphs. To do that, I need to, at the risk of testing your patience, distinguish between two sorts of monocularity.

The sort of monocularity I mentioned in the preceding section grows out of the natural tendency to conserve mental energy, and it is a sign of intellectual lassitude (or, sometimes, political expediency). The second sort of monocularity, however, grows out of moral integrity, specifically, out of a commitment to act. That is, it is important to recognize the respect in which, when we act, we have to stop using two lenses. We can't choose to get and not get the same intervention aimed at improvement. To the extent that binocular thinking can impede action, it is plainly morally undesirable. This book's two epigraphs are supposed to flag the fundamental and fertile tension between the two goals of better thinking and better action, between the aspiration to achieve binocularity and the recognition of the need to accept temporary monocularity of the second sort.

The first epigraph is supposed to remind us of that first goal: better thinking. According to the 8th-century c.e. Buddhist, Sen-ts'an, those who profess to love truth need to resist choosing sides: "If you want the truth to stand clear before you, never be for or against. The struggle between 'for' and 'against' is the mind's worst disease."[14] Rather than choose between lenses, the binocular aspiration is to use both.

The second epigraph—the title of a civil rights song, "Which Side Are You On?"—is supposed to remind us of that second goal: acting better. It is supposed to remind those who profess to love justice that sometimes we have to choose sides and lenses. In this sense, the pursuit of justice can, at least temporarily, require monocularity. Again, though, if using one lens at the end of a binocular process is a form of monocularity, it is monocularity born of moral integrity, not intellectual laziness. It is reasonable, I think, to consider that a monocular moment in a binocular process.

A MORE BINOCULAR HABIT OF THINKING ABOUT INFORMED CONSENT

I will have to wait until chapter 7 to become more explicit about what such a process would entail. There I will consider one relatively specific instance of technologically shaping our selves: the process of families and professionals making decisions about whether to use surgery to normalize the appearance of children with atypical bodies. In my description of a binocular habit of thinking about the process of truly informed consent, it will quickly become evident how a binocular habit of comprehending persons can be useful: since, as objects, our preferences are constituted by myriad social and biological forces beneath or beyond our awareness, it is our responsibility to reflect on those forces— whether they initially make us prone to refuse or to request surgical intervention. That is, on my account, in the first stage of the informed-consent process, we show respect to the person who will live with the consequences of the decision by treating her as an object—*in the sense that* we challenge her to consider the forces bearing down on her. To facilitate that challenge, we invite her to oscillate between the stances and lenses that inevitably arise in the context of such decisions. In the context of appearance-normalizing surgeries, for example, we will discover the value of oscillating between the so-called medical and social lenses through which we can consider the meaning of having an atypical body.

And, except in those rare cases where patients demonstrate that they are incapable of making an informed choice, in the second stage of the process, medical professionals have a responsibility to treat patients as subjects, who can freely choose. In this stage of the process, the professional defers to the patient's truly informed choice, whether the choice is to refuse or request intervention. It is by deferring to others' choices, which we might not make for ourselves, that we show respect for patients as subjects.

A METAPHOR, NOT A SYSTEM

So, because we understand the respect in which we are all objects whose preferences are determined by myriad biological and social forces, we aspire to engage in explicitly binocular thinking in the first stage of the informed-consent process. That is, we aspire to help the person who is making the decision to oscillate between the stances of the critics of intervention and the enthusiasts about intervention, and between the conceptual lenses that the competing sides offer. For the sake of action, however, such binocular thinking has to stop. In the second stage of the process, we treat persons as subjects, and we defer to their choices. The good news here is that, even though the explicitly binocular thinking comes to a stop, the process as a whole is binocular, insofar as it reflects a binocular understanding of persons.

At all costs, though, I want to avoid the appearance of suffering from the delusion that I have a system for thinking about technologically shaping our selves. I do not. I intend the metaphor of binocularity to suggest a habit of thinking, which can help make our understanding deeper and our actions better—and which not only recognizes, but embraces, the tension between those two aspirations. I will consider myself successful if I can begin to describe a habit of thinking that is more fruitful than the one I brought to the debates those many years ago, when, as I described in chapter 1, I tried to win the argument against enhancement rather than try to understand what it means.

Chapter 3

Creativity and Gratitude

In the preceding chapter I distinguished between large and small binary choices. The conclusion that, for example, one is for or against enhancement entails a big binary choice, and defending that conclusion then requires many smaller ones, such as between emphasizing that persons are subjects who are free and emphasizing that persons are objects whose actions are determined. In this chapter I describe in some detail what I call the "stances" from which the conclusion for or against enhancement can feel right, and I suggest that only by oscillating between those stances can we achieve a deeper comprehension of the meaning of enhancement. Finally, I describe more briefly some more of the conceptual "lenses" that we sometimes imagine we have to—but don't really have to—choose between when we're after deeper comprehension.

As with the term *stance*, with the term *lens* I am emphasizing that what we see in these debates is always partial, in the sense that they give us only incomplete comprehension and in the sense that they are skewed in a way that feels right to us. A more binocular habit of thinking entails remembering that partiality and also waiting for as long as possible to make the large and small binary choices that the debates about technologically shaping our selves constantly invite us to make. It aspires to resist the sort of monocularity that we can settle into when winning a point matters more than understanding what's at issue.

ACADEMIC HEAT

The debates about enhancement in the United States and United Kingdom have at times been intense. Some critics have suggested that their opponents have shallow souls[1] or are paving the way for new guillotines or gas chambers.[2] Some enthusiasts have suggested that their opponents have stunted powers of rational analysis[3] or secretly hope to establish a theocracy,[4] which seems to put newcomers to the debates in the unenviable position of having to choose to side with either devils or idiots.

I speculate that, to some extent, the intensity of the enhancement debate can be explained by the fact that, when we argue for our side, it can feel like we are doing no less than arguing for the value of our own existence, justifying our way of being in the world. If, to take a not terribly far-fetched example, I am by nature-nurture prone to melancholy and slowness and appreciation of the world as we find it, I am unlikely to argue vigorously for the superiority of high spirits, speed, and the creative transformation of the world. If you are by nature-nurture prone to high spirits, speed, and transformation of the world as we find it, you are unlikely to argue for the superiority of the alternatives.

For most of human history, human beings did not have to justify their own ways of being. The serf didn't take himself to have chosen serfdom any more than the king chose to be king. Those roles were ordained by God or Fate or Nature. We children of modernity, however, tend to think that we have chosen our own ways of being, and thus we feel the burden of justifying our choice.[5]

Unfortunately, the language we use to justify our own ways of being depends on a vast network of binary oppositions. They invite us to imagine that to grasp the nature of whatever is at hand, we have to choose one pole *or* the other of a given opposition—even when a moment's thought reveals that both poles emphasize different but equally salient features of the same phenomenon. We find ourselves in an intellectual double bind: first our thinking is constrained by our desire to justify our own way of being, and then by the fact that, to articulate that self-justification, we have to choose between the poles of various binary oppositions. The very sorts of psychological capacity and linguistic structure that are the necessary conditions for the pursuit of understanding can conspire against it.

THE MORAL IDEAL OF AUTHENTICITY

The work of the philosopher Charles Taylor helps to make conspicuous our tendency to accept the sorts of big and small binary choices that we would refuse to make if it was understanding that we were after. In particular, I have in mind Taylor's account of the debates between what he calls the "knockers and boosters of modernity"—especially his observation that the two sides of that debate fail to recognize the fundamental moral ideal that they share: the moral ideal of authenticity.[6] Before beginning to suggest a way in which the critics of and enthusiasts about technologically shaping our selves similarly fail, however, I should clarify what Taylor means by "the knockers and boosters of modernity."

According to him, much of the debate between the knockers and boosters of modernity, a debate that is very much with us today, is rooted in each side's different mistake about the same moral ideal. The moral ideal of authenticity, which he says emerged fully at the end of the eighteenth century in Europe, is that each of us should find our own way of being in the world. It is my job as a human being to find my way of flourishing, of being true to myself. "If I am not [true to myself], I miss the point of my life, I miss what being human is for me."[7]

To understand Taylor—and, as I will explain below, I think he has been misunderstood by some participants in the enhancement debates—it is imperative to understand what he means when he says that the debate about the moral ideal of authenticity is "inarticulate." We need to understand what he means when he, somewhat enigmatically, says of the ideal: "Its opponents slight it, and its friends can't speak of it."[8]

When Taylor wrote *The Ethics of Authenticity*, Allan Bloom's *The Closing of the American Mind* was being widely discussed, and Bloom became Taylor's paradigmatic "knocker" of modernity. Much of *Closing of the American Mind* lambastes American college students and their teachers for their self-indulgence and shallowness, which Bloom says they cloak in "a certain rhetoric of self-fulfillment."[9] What Bloom doesn't understand, according to Taylor, is that, even if some students and their teachers are guilty of self-indulgence and shallowness, many in fact are striving to live up to the moral ideal of authenticity. Whether or not they achieve it, they aspire to find self-fulfillment, to become who they really are. That is, where Bloom sees rampant immorality, Taylor sees a powerful moral ideal at work. Bloom fails to see the robustness of the conception of a good life at work in the pursuit of self-fulfillment.

Taylor doesn't, however, think that only the knockers of modernity fail to appreciate the robustness or thickness of the moral ideal of authenticity. He thinks the boosters make the same mistake, if from the opposite direction. Their mistake, he suggests, is built into what he calls "the liberalism of neutrality."[10] He suggests that this variety of liberalism has as one of its basic tenets "that a liberal society must be neutral on questions of what constitutes a good life."[11] To put Taylor's point even more bluntly than he does in *The Ethics of Authenticity* (or in *Sources of the Self*), there is an important respect in which no theory about living well together can be neutral about what constitutes a good life. Such a theory requires a conception of what is good the way seeing requires a horizon. Theories about living well together can be set against different horizons, but they cannot do without one, no matter how fervently we wish it were otherwise.

In a nutshell, Taylor thinks the boosters of modernity fail to recognize that the moral ideal of authenticity is tacitly at work in the liberalism of neutrality. They fail to notice that, insofar as the liberalism of neutrality is committed to affirming persons in their own projects of self-fulfillment, it is not neutral. In our commitment to refraining from specifying the forms of self-fulfillment that individuals should pursue, we liberals forget the way our commitment to self-fulfillment itself instantiates a conception of the good life. It's just that this view of the good life is so ubiquitous that it doesn't seem like a *moral* ideal; it seems like just what every reasonable person desires.

CRITICS OF, AND ENTHUSIASTS ABOUT, ENHANCEMENT

Again, Taylor is not talking in *The Ethics of Authenticity* about the debate over so-called enhancement technologies in particular or technologically shaping selves in general. (He is talking about "relativism.") I offer his account of the debates between the knockers and boosters of modernity to suggest a way of understanding the debates between the critics of and enthusiasts about enhancement and, ultimately, about technologically shaping our selves in general. Namely, I want to suggest that the critics of enhancement tend to "slight" the moral ideal that can be at work in efforts at technological self-transformation and that the enthusiasts "can't speak of," or recognize the robustness of, the moral ideal at work in their exhortation to create our own life projects. In more positive terms, I want to suggest that the knockers and boosters of—or critics of and enthusiasts about—"enhancement technologies" share the moral ideal of authenticity, but they emphasize different insights regarding what it means, and thus about how to achieve it. They share the same fundamental moral ideal but see it from such different stances and through such different lenses that it is hard for them to remember what they share.

Some participants in the bioethical debates about enhancement have, I believe, misunderstood Charles Taylor to be endorsing the sort of criticism of enhancement that can be found in the philosopher Carl Elliott's work,[12] perhaps because Elliott brought Taylor's discussion of authenticity to the enhancement debates. That is, those participants mistakenly trace a critical view of enhancement to Taylor. The philosopher Neil Levy, for example, suggests that we should consider Jean-Paul Sartre's conception of authenticity and enthusiasm for self-shaping as an alternative to what he takes to be Taylor's criticism.[13] In fact, Taylor's primary aim is to persuade us that we should refuse to choose between the "knockers" and "boosters" of modernity and authenticity, just as I am urging us to refuse to choose between the critics of and enthusiasts about enhancement (and as I think Levy, too, ultimately urges us to do).[14] I could not agree more with Taylor than when he says that we need to get over arguing for or against authenticity and that we need to talk *about* what it means.[15]

THE CRITICS' CONCERN THAT ENHANCEMENT
THREATENS AUTHENTICITY

When critics articulate concerns about enhancement, one of their core ones is that its pursuit will entail the loss of authenticity or the threat of alienation. They worry that a given technological intervention will separate us from who we really are or from what is most our own: our own way of flourishing. Even if the term *authenticity* (or *alienation*) is not always explicit, the concept usually is. Sometimes, however, the concept and term are explicit, and nowhere more than in the widely cited report *Beyond Therapy*, which was written by George W. Bush's President's Council on Bioethics.[16] In that report, Leon Kass and the members of the council speak at length about mood-altering drugs like Prozac, among other examples. In a word, they worry that mood-altering drugs will separate us from the actions and experiences that normally accompany our moods. They worry that in becoming separated from those un-drug-mediated experiences, we will be separated from who we really are and from how the world really is. They write, "As the power to transform our native powers increases, both in magnitude and refinement, so does the possibility for 'self-alienation'—for losing, confounding, or abandoning our identity."[17]

Some participant observers in the enhancement debates, from both the enthusiastic[18] and critical[19] camps, have suggested that the debate between critics and enthusiasts is one more instance of traditional debates between political conservatives and liberals, with liberals being enthusiastic and conservatives being critical. The fact that the President's Council, led by a political conservative, invoked the language of authenticity to criticize enhancement may seem to support that suggestion. We should notice, however, the extent to which that suggestion terribly simplifies a complex intellectual terrain. The difference between critics and enthusiasts is simply not the same as the difference between political "conservatives" and "progressives."[20] In fact, some of the most astute and eloquent critics of enhancement are political progressives.[21]

PROGRESSIVE CRITICS WORRY WE WILL BECOME SEPARATED FROM WHO WE REALLY ARE

There is perhaps no more eloquent or progressive a critic of technologically shaping selves than Carl Elliott. In his book *Better Than Well*,[22] Elliott advances an important claim that is familiar to political progressives: the medical-industrial complex creates desires in us for stuff we don't need. While one of his concerns is about how the medical-industrial complex shamelessly uses the rhetoric of authenticity to hawk its wares, his primary concern is that those wares will make us different from who we really are. As he puts it in *Better Than Well*,

> Many enhancement technologies are ... [unsettling] ... not primarily because they enhance people, but because they affect something central to their identities.... What is at issue is not simply whether the change is for the better or for the worse ... *but the mere fact that the person has changed* [emphasis added].[23]

Elliott's concern is that such products will make us different from who we really are or separate us from who we really are; they will make us inauthentic.

As a progressive intellectual, he is keenly aware that relying on any notion of an authentic self can sound perilously close to outré notions like "the essential self" or "the real self." Though Elliott is as wary as anyone about conceptions of an essential self—if that phrase entails any commitment to a belief in an essence given by God or Nature—he rightly thinks that we can and do talk about authenticity without any such commitment, and he offers innumerable examples in his book.

PROGRESSIVE CRITICS WORRY WE WILL BECOME SEPARATED FROM THE WORLD AS IT REALLY IS

There is a sense, though, in which Elliott's concern in particular and the critics' concern more generally are less about the state of the self than about the state of the relationship between the self and the social world. When Elliott worries about technologies like Prozac, he worries that they will separate us from what is most our own—where what is most our own is a true relationship to the world as it really is. We might say his deepest worry is that such a drug will alienate us from our alienation, that it will separate us from the ways in which the world really is alienating. Indeed, if a downside of Elliott's view is that it can sometimes seem insensitive to the suffering of real human beings who want to avail themselves of a technology to reduce their suffering in the social world as it is, one of the most compelling and important things about Elliott's critique is that it takes so seriously the individual's relationship to the social world.

I hasten to add that, when Elliott worries about Prozac, he isn't worried about it as a treatment for clinical depression, if by clinical depression we refer to a cluster of symptoms that are disproportionate responses to the world as it is. Rather, for Elliott, Prozac is a proxy for some future drug that could eliminate a painful but proportionate response to the world as it is.

Perhaps even more explicitly than in *Better Than Well*, in an earlier essay,[24] Elliott expressed his worry about a drug that might separate us from the world as it really is. There he invented a character, an accountant living in Downers Grove, Illinois, who comes to himself one day and says, "Jesus Christ, is this it? A Snapper lawn mower and a house in the suburbs?" Elliott invites us to imagine that we are this man's psychiatrist. Should we prescribe Prozac? Or should we think that, "even though he's in a predicament, at least he's aware of it, which is a lot better than being in a predicament and thinking you're not"?[25]

Elliott traces this idea about the value of knowing you're in a predicament to the novelist Walker Percy,[26] who traces the same idea to Søren Kierkegaard,[27] one of the progenitors of the notion of authenticity. According to all three, failing to recognize that you are in a predicament—that you are dis-eased—is the worst disease of all. Turning away from one's despair—becoming separated from the alienation that is proportionate to the character of the world as it is—is what worries Elliott (and the other critics). He worries about any intervention that would separate us from how the world really is and, insofar as who we are is constituted by our relationship to the world, would also separate us from who we really are.

ENTHUSIASTS HOPE ENHANCEMENTS PROMOTE AUTHENTICITY

Enthusiasts about enhancement, of course, see these same technologies very differently. But it's crucial to notice that enthusiasts, too, are committed to the moral ideal of authenticity. Much of Peter Kramer's *Listening to Prozac* aims to allay the sort of worry about the loss of authenticity that can be found in Kierkegaard, Percy, and Elliott. Kramer argues that drugs like Prozac can actually give us what is most our own, that they can free us to encounter the world as it really is, in all of its difficulty. On his view, Prozac doesn't rob life of the edifying potential for tragedy but rather "catalyzes the precondition for tragedy, namely, participation."[28]

In the same spirit, the philosopher David DeGrazia[29] invites his readers to consider the case of a young woman who had a traumatic childhood, who isn't leading the life she imagines for herself, and who asks her doctor to prescribe Prozac so that she can transform herself. Against those who would criticize this young woman's request, DeGrazia writes, "It is hard to see the basis of paternalistically judging that her values and self-conception are not authoritative for her own life—not only for what is good in her life (best interests) but also for what constitutes her life (authenticity). I therefore conclude that Prozac... can be an authentic part of a project of self-creation."[30] DeGrazia is suggesting that, rather than alienate this young woman from her self, Prozac allows her to become who she really is. It allows her to craft her own life project as she envisions it; it facilitates her project of self-creation.

I should point out that, in addition to, and sometimes together with, the metaphor of self-*creation*, enthusiasts also sometimes use the metaphor of self-*recovery* or self-*discovery* when they give their account of how enhancement technologies can promote authenticity. To quickly see how the metaphors of self-creation and self-discovery can work together to support the argument for Prozac as a tool to promote authenticity, we need look no farther than an advertisement for Prozac's chemical sibling, Paxil, which appeared in a medical journal many years ago.

To grasp the ad's moral argument, one needs to remember Michelangelo's famous claim that his sculptures were already there in the marble and that his task was merely to chip away at the excess that stood between him and the sculpture he found. According to this way of speaking, he didn't create the sculpture so much as he discovered, or recovered, it.

The Paxil ad has two parts, with the first taking up one page and the second part taking up two. The first line of the ad reads: "The imprisoned patient." Most of the page is taken up with a picture of an unfinished sculpture of a man who appears to be trying to break out of the excess marble that imprisons him. (Indeed, the glossy ad makes a direct allusion to Michelangelo's statue, *The Prisoner*, which he never finished, due to a labor dispute with his employer, the Pope.)

Across the top of the next two pages of the ad is a sculptor's chisel, emblazoned with the word PAXIL. At the very end of the ad is a picture of the formerly imprisoned patient, who now holds his arms up toward the sky, exultant in his newfound freedom. Paxil is the tool that allowed the true, free, authentic self to emerge. According to the ad's argument, like Michelangelo, the psychiatrist *re-* or *dis-covers*—and sets free—the true self, the self that was there all along. And, insofar as the psychiatrist is the artist who wields the chisel that is Paxil, she is also the *creator* of the new, free, authentic self. The metaphors of creation and discovery are used together to advance the enthusiast's case for intervention.

All of which is to say that the disagreement between critics and enthusiasts isn't about whether authenticity is an important moral ideal, but about what fulfilling that ideal entails, and about whether a given intervention will thwart or promote someone's efforts to achieve it.

THE UBIQUITY OF THE LANGUAGE OF AUTHENTICITY

It is hard to exaggerate the extent to which we, in our efforts to justify our ways of being, repair to the language of authenticity, whether we are criticizing or endorsing the use of new technologies to shape our selves. When, for example, people who can't hear justify their refusal of a technological intervention that would allow them to hear, they emphasize that deafness, and the culture that has grown up around that anatomical difference, is an essential feature of who they are.[31] That is why they demand to be called Deaf, with a capital "d." They reject cochlear implants, at least in part, on the grounds that the interventions would keep them from being who they really are.

Conversely, when people who can't hear justify their choice to get cochlear implants, they say that the intervention will allow them to become whole, more fully human, authentic. As Michael Chorost, who was born hard of hearing and became completely deaf in his thirties, put it in his book *Rebuilt: How Becoming Part Computer Made Me More Human*: "What saved me from alienation was not just being able to hear again, but also being forced to construct my world rather than simply taking it as given."[32] In the penultimate sentence of his narrative, he says that once he got his cochlear implant, he could finally walk out his door "and encounter the world whole and full."[33] Different from the Paxil advertisers, Chorost does not say that he and his audiologist uncovered the self or the world as they always were there, but, like the Paxil advertisers, he suggests that using the technology set him free. The cochlear implants were the chisel he used to creatively construct his world and, in so doing, to overcome alienation and achieve authenticity.

If, for example, a woman wants to explain why she doesn't want a breast enlargement (or reduction) she can say that such an intervention would make her different from who she really is. And if a woman wants to explain why she wants such an intervention, she can say that the intervention will allow others to finally discover who she really is under the misleading exterior. To her surprise, when the feminist sociologist Kathy Davis interviewed thoughtful women in the early 1990s who decided to get such surgeries, they all reported a similar experience: each had a body part that "just didn't belong."[34] That body part, according to Davis, was perceived by each woman "as an alien (and alienating) encumbrance which transformed her body so that it did not correspond to who she 'really' was."[35]

On my reading of Ilina Singh's ethnographic research on children diagnosed with Attention-Deficit Hyperactivity Disorder (ADHD),[36] children, too, speak the language of authenticity: those who think they don't benefit from pharmacological treatment say it makes them different from who they really are, while those (the majority of her subjects) who think they do benefit from the intervention say it doesn't make them different from who they really are. They say it enables their capacity for moral agency. On such an account, the drugs used to treat ADHD don't enslave children but liberate them.

Much the same goes for adult poets when they talk about the experience of taking antidepressants: the ones who think it isn't beneficial say it separates them from who they really are, and the ones who think it is beneficial say it removes a barrier between themselves and their work; they say it enables them to do their work.[37] People who want to get and those who want to refuse treatment for anorexia are equally adept at deploying the language of authenticity.[38] While people with healthy limbs aren't very often called on to justify their preference to retain them, people who desire to have healthy limbs removed say that's the only way they can become who they really are.[39] They are wont to say removing their healthy limbs is the only way they can become "whole."[40] And in the case of transgender surgery and pharmacology, there is the long-standing disagreement between those who suggest that such interventions entail a denial of one's true, norm-challenging self,[41] and those who suggest that it is only by way of such interventions that they can become who they really are.[42]

So critics and enthusiasts both can invoke (whether explicitly or tacitly) the moral ideal of authenticity to support their stance. Critics claim that a given technological intervention will separate us from who we really are, and enthusiasts claim the same intervention will enable or facilitate our becoming who we really are. This state of affairs is puzzling, however, only if we fall into the trap of reification—only if we forget that authenticity is not a thing, but a moral ideal. When we forget that authenticity is an abstract moral ideal, we become vulnerable to thinking that one side can be right (and thus the other wrong) about whether a given intervention will promote "it." That trap is as easy to fall into as it is hugely important to try to avoid.

THE CREATIVITY AND GRATITUDE
STANCES

When the enthusiast James Hughes referred in his book *Citizen Cyborg* to the critics of enhancement, he called them "Bioluddites."[43] The people who disagreed with him were backward-looking reactionaries, with nothing insightful to say about the nature of human beings or human flourishing. By contrast, those on his side of the debate were "transhumanists," a label he took to have a positive valence and to describe those with the intellectual and moral courage to look forward and embrace the future.

When one of the most widely read critics, Michael Sandel, on the other hand, referred to the enthusiasts, he said they proceeded to the debate from an "ethic of willfulness."[44] Those who disagreed with him were modern-day Prometheans: gluttons for technological power, insensitive to its true moral cost. By contrast, he said that those on his side of the debate proceeded from an "ethic of giftedness"[45]—a label he took to have a positive valence.

By suggesting above that the two sides proceed to the debate from different but equally ethical interpretations of the same moral ideal of authenticity, I began to indicate what I think is wrong with understanding the debate in terms of "we insightful ones" against "those obtuse ones," or we good ones against those evil ones, or we rational ones against those emotional ones. My sense of the unhelpfulness of those labels has driven me to look for an alternative pair of labels, both of which would have a positive valence and which thus would signal that potentially complementary insights are at work on both sides.

In the past I have suggested *creativity* as a positively valenced label for the stance that the enthusiasts tend to feel most comfortable adopting. In the creativity stance, the human capacity to creatively transform ourselves and the world feels worthy of celebration. From this stance, human beings are by nature "creators." They are agents, who have the capacity to create themselves. That is, those who speak from the creativity stance are speaking from a deep, but particular, human anthropology, or conception of the nature of human beings. Neil Levy sums up that anthropology, when he writes:

> We are … animals of a peculiar sort: we are self-creating and self-modifying animals. … The sciences of the mind offer us new opportunities for altering our minds and increasing their powers, but in so doing they offer us new means of doing what we have always done; the kind of thing that *makes us the beings that we are* [emphasis added].[46]

Levy's interpretation regarding the nature of human beings gives support to his generally enthusiastic stance toward using new technologies to shape our selves. On the enthusiastic interpretation, to creatively transform our selves is to act in accordance with our natures. And at least since Aristotle, we in the West have thought that acting in accordance with our natures is precisely what we ought to try to do. That is, what we understand the nature of humans to be (our "anthropologies") is intimately connected to how we think we ought to act (our ethics). For those proceeding from what I'm calling the creativity stance, we have, as human beings, an ethical responsibility to creatively transform our selves and the world.

In the past I have suggested *gratitude* as a positively valenced label for the stance that critics tend to find congenial. In the gratitude stance, the human capacity to recognize that we have been thrown into being by forces we don't yet understand and that we didn't create feels worthy of celebration. In this stance, we recognize the respect in which we are objects; we didn't throw ourselves into being. In other words, from the gratitude stance, we are by nature "creatures." Life is not something we have created or earned or deserve, but it is "a gift." As a gift, we should accept and affirm it. We should learn to let things be, to be slower to transform them to meet our passing desires. As Michael Sandel puts it, "To acknowledge the giftedness of life is to recognize that our talents and powers are not wholly our own doing, nor even fully ours, despite the efforts we expend to develop and exercise them. It is also to recognize that not everything in the world is open to any use we may desire or devise."[47] As for the enthusiasts, for the critics, too, there is an important connection between their anthropologies (we are creatures, for whom life is a gift) and their ethics (we should be cautious in, as it were, transforming that gift).

BOTH STANCES CAN BE TRACED TO "RELIGIOUS" ROOTS

It was not surprising to me to learn that the term *gratitude* does not have a positive valence for many enthusiasts. To begin with, they often suggest that the exhortation to "affirm what is given" is on its face at best foolish. After all, along with our lives, we have been given tuberculosis and Tay-Sachs and cancer and tsunamis and tornados and volcanoes. I think, though, that here the enthusiast fails to hear what the critic is trying to say when she invokes the value of affirming what is. The critic cannot be, and is not, saying that we should affirm *everything*—any more than a thoughtful enthusiast would say we should creatively transform *everything*. She is saying that there is goodness in more ways of being than we are prone to notice when we look at our selves from the creativity stance. She is saying that, were we to notice that goodness, we would squander less energy on transforming human bodies to conform to unduly narrow conceptions of how to be. The critic's point isn't that creative self-transformation is inherently bad but that letting our selves be can be good.[48]

It has been more surprising to me to notice that this term *gratitude*, which I intend to have a positive valence, can also have a negative valence for many critics. The simple reason, of course, is that the notion of life as a gift can seem to entail the profession of knowledge of a Giver—specifically, of the God of organized religion. Frankly, as someone who does not practice an organized religion and who is deeply discomfited by all claims to knowledge of God, that reason seems to me to be very bad, if not paranoid. It simply is not true that emphasizing the respect in which life is a gift requires professing any knowledge at all of any sort of Giver.[49] To talk about life as a gift is to signal one's awareness of the simple but fundamental fact that we did not create our selves or the world. It could have been otherwise: there could have been no us and no world, but there are both. Surely Socrates, for whom "awe and wonder" were the beginning of philosophy, did not profess knowledge of the source of humankind or the world. In comparison to Socrates's contempt for those who did profess such knowledge, Richard Dawkins, Daniel Dennett, Sam Harris, and Christopher Hitchens are pikers.[50]

Instead of using the label *gratitude*, I could use another label, such as "acceptance" or "appreciation."[51] Again, I, of course, understand that I live in a culture where some of us build our identities on our embrace—or rejection—of organized religion. So I understand that by avoiding the term *gratitude* I would avoid any religious associations and thereby avoid the risk of saying something that could be construed as relevant for those identities. In fact,

I prefer *gratitude* because it does not attempt to erase the religious association, but it instead reminds us of an important, underappreciated feature of the enhancement debates in particular and the debates about technologically shaping selves more generally. I want to use the label *gratitude* and the label *creativity* precisely because both terms can help remind us of some ancient sources of our competing interpretations of, and intuitions regarding, how human beings are and ought to be.

That is, just as it isn't only the critics who are saddled with a commitment to the moral ideal of authenticity, it isn't only the critics whose fundamental insight regarding the nature of human beings has "religious roots." Yes, it is true that one of the Ur-critics of enhancement was the Protestant theologian Paul Ramsey, who argued that, lest we become inhumane, we must remember that we are *creatures of* God.[52] It is every bit as true, however, that one of the Ur-enthusiasts was also a Protestant theologian. Joseph Fletcher argued—against the stereotype clung to by some enthusiasts—that human beings have an ethical obligation to use technology to improve the world; on such an account, human beings are meant to be *co-creators with* God.[53] Fletcher is not an outlier. The idea of human beings, together with God, co-creating or perfecting the universe has deep roots in Christianity and Judaism.

Theologically inclined critics can appeal to one strand of their traditions to support an anthropology of creatureliness, and theologically inclined enthusiasts can appeal to another strand of the same traditions to support an anthropology of creativity. The difference between the two sides isn't that one appeals to an idea with religious roots and the other doesn't. The difference is that one side emphasizes one insight with religious roots and the other side another. Deep, ancient insights and intuitions regarding the nature of human beings and regarding our proper relationship to our selves and the world are at work on both sides.

CONCEPTUAL CHOICES
NO ONE WHO LOVED TRUTH
SHOULD BE WILLING TO MAKE

We have just noticed that critics tend to be comfortable in one stance, or general attitude, toward ourselves and the world, and enthusiasts tend to be comfortable in a different, though complementary, one: the critics are partial to letting our selves and the world be, and the enthusiasts are partial to creatively transforming our selves and the world. Of course, that isn't to say that people on the two sides adopt only one stance. As most wisdom traditions would remind us, the key is in finding some sort of balance between them. But in the heat of academic battle, we tend to forget the aspiration to balance, and we tend to speak from the stance we find most congenial.

We also just noticed that the stance toward our selves and the world that we are partial to affects which conceptual lenses we are partial to. Whereas, for example, people who are most comfortable in the gratitude stance tend to be comfortable using the lens through which we see human beings as creatures, people most comfortable in the creativity stance tend to be comfortable using the lens through which we see human beings as creators. Each of those conceptual lenses allows us to see something enormously important, but neither of them can by itself let us see in depth.

Of course when we're trying to make the case for or against technological intervention, we won't need to use one lens only. To make a case from either stance, we need to draw on insights from clusters of lenses. In the next chapter, I will describe in some detail the opposing lenses through which critics and enthusiasts see what technology is. Here I want to just mention a few other examples of pairs of lenses that we sometimes imagine we have to choose between, even though we surely don't—and shouldn't.

When, for example, the enthusiast Julian Savulescu argues for using new technologies to enhance athletic performance, he says that what distinguishes "human sport...from animal sport" is that the former is "creative." He elaborates what he thinks epitomizes human sport when he writes, "Biological manipulation embodies the human spirit—the capacity to improve ourselves on the basis of reasons and judgment. *When we exercise our reason, we do what only humans do*" (emphasis added).[54] That is, on the enthusiast's view, what is most distinctive about human beings is our creativity, which here refers to our ability to use *reason* to achieve control and exercise power over our selves to improve them.

When, however, the bioethicist Tom Murray builds a case against enhancement, he emphasizes our creatureliness, the ways in which our lives are contingent and we are vulnerable.[55] As he puts it, the problem with the pursuit of enhancement is that it is "spurred by a desire to escape the limitations and especially the hurts that mark indelibly our existence as finite, embodied, interdependent beings."[56] For Murray, it is in *emotional* relationships (especially those formed in families)—not in an individual's exercise of reason to exert control—that we glimpse the feature of ourselves that is most distinctive and marvelous. It's not that Murray denies the salience of reason, power, control, or independence. Rather, he fears that in the pursuit of what Savulescu calls enhancement, we will lose sight of those features of our being that most deserve preservation, including emotion, vulnerability, mutuality, and interdependence.

This thread in the enhancement debate, which emphasizes that we should affirm our vulnerability and embodiedness, is nowhere easier to glimpse than in the work of the philosopher Hans Jonas, who argues that our vulnerability—in particular the fact that we will die—is not only a gigantic burden, but, as he puts it, also a great blessing. Grappling with the prospect of death, he avers, is an essential part of living well:

> Only in confrontation with ever-possible not-being could being come to feel itself, affirm itself, make itself its own purpose.... The gain [of the sense of subjectivity] is double edged like every trait of life. Feeling lies open to pain as well as to pleasure, its keenness cutting both ways; lust has its match in anguish, desire in fear; purpose is either attained or thwarted, and the capacity for enjoying the one is the same as suffering from the other.[57]

Critics of enhancement are quick to make this point about the double-edgedness of our traits. Sometimes they invoke a simple fact like the one that the gene variant associated with sickle cell anemia also protects against malaria. More ambitiously, a writer like Joshua Wolf Shenk argues that Abraham Lincoln's depression was not only a gigantic burden and source of suffering, but also an essential ingredient in his great life.[58] This notion that we can't extricate what is hardest about being animals like us without doing damage to what is greatest or most important is a recurrent theme among the critics.

Critics tend to see human beings as organisms: staggeringly complex and fragile systems, which, like the rest of the natural world, are easy to harm and devilishly hard to improve. In this sense, critics see us through an "ecological" lens. Enthusiasts, on the other hand, tend to be partial to using an "engineering" lens.[59] Through the engineering lens, human beings, and the rest of the natural world, look like complex machines that, with enough techno-scientific progress, we can shape to meet our desires.

One enthusiast is so sanguine about our emerging understanding of that machinery that he suggests we have an ethical obligation to engineer all suffering out of all human and nonhuman animals.[60] Though surely not nearly that sanguine about the prospect of extirpating human suffering, Peter Kramer suggested, in his second book about depression, that we might one day use gene-transfer technology to remove the sort of alienation that is humanly useless, while preserving the sort that is useful.[61] More recently Allen Buchanan has adduced facts about the modularity of human traits, which he takes to suggest that the engineering project is much more doable than the ecological-lens-wielding critics assume.[62]

The enthusiasts' confidence in our ability to engineer such traits seems to me actually out of step with many recent advances in the genetics and neuroscience of complex behaviors, but that is an empirical question.[63] My simple conceptual point is that the ecological and engineering lenses are different, important, and at work in, respectively, the gratitude and creativity stances.

CONCLUSION

The heat of academic battle about technologically shaping our selves can make us forget that, while most of us feel more comfortable in the gratitude stance or in the creativity stance, none of us feels comfortable in only one. Oscillating between the stances and the lenses associated with them comes naturally to thoughtful people, even if acknowledging such oscillation sometimes doesn't. Moreover, the heat of academic battle can make us forget that we share a commitment to the moral ideal of authenticity (whether or not we explicitly use or like that term). In such forgetfulness, in the pursuit of winning the point or justifying our selves, we become hypervulnerable to making the sorts of conceptual choices that our language keeps inviting us to make, and that we would refuse to make if deeper comprehension were our aim.

In a cooler context, we would refuse to choose between thinking of persons as creators or creatures, just as we would refuse to think of them as essentially reasonable or essentially emotional. We would refuse to choose between thinking that suffering is the always-to-be-extirpated enemy or that it is the always-to-be-welcomed source of growth. We would also refuse to choose between understanding our selves as engineerable mechanisms or as fragile ecological webs. In the next chapter I suggest that we need to get over making similarly unhelpful choices, if we are trying to understand what technology is and when we should use it.

Chapter 4

Technology as Value-Free
and as Value-Laden

As I mentioned in chapter 1, my initial conclusion regarding enhancement was that it was bad. And, as I suggested in the preceding chapter, I have come to understand the extent to which that conclusion was a predictable outgrowth of the stance toward the world that I feel most comfortable in and have called "the gratitude stance." However, in the early and mid-1990s, when I attempted to defend my conclusion in academic debate, I didn't mention anything about the role of feeling in, or about the partiality of, my view. The enthusiasts, whom I now take to have been speaking from what I have called "the creativity stance," seemed to be claiming that they had gotten over feeling and partiality and were speaking from reason alone, so I tried to speak as if I thought I was doing the same.

A key element in that argument against enhancement and other forms of technologically shaping our selves was my observation that "means matter morally."[1] I spent a lot of time arguing that it makes an ethical difference whether we use technological or nontechnological means to achieve a given end or purpose. I tried to say why, for example, it might be good to help a student improve her classroom performance with a nontechnological means like increasing her engagement with her teacher, but it might be bad to achieve the same end with a technological means like medication. I suggested that, for example, whereas a technological means like medication expressed or emphasized values like efficiency, speed, and control, a nontechnological means like increasing teacher-student interaction expressed or emphasized values like engagement, slowness, and affirming different ways of being a student.

I still think it's deeply important to consider how means matter morally, but I want to give up the "monocular" approach I adopted when trying to win the point. In this chapter I want to suggest the usefulness of understanding what technology is in at least two ways, which at first seem incompatible. Through the lens that is ready at hand in the creativity stance, technology is value-free (or morally neutral) and we use it to shape ourselves as we see fit. Through the lens that is ready at hand in the gratitude stance, technology is value-laden and it shapes us in ways that usually elude our attention. A more binocular understanding of technology benefits from the insights that are visible through both lenses.

THE ENTANGLEMENT OF IS AND OUGHT

The debate between enthusiasts and critics isn't complicated only because they use different lenses for understanding what technology is. It is further complicated because their different understandings of what technology is either presuppose, or are presupposed by, their different understandings of what nature is and what human nature is. As we will see, the critics' and enthusiasts' different understandings of those concepts (and, as we saw in the previous chapter, their understandings of other concepts, too) do, at least temporarily, cluster in predictable ways. Some lenses have, as it were, natural affinities for each other.

I am emphasizing, again, that what both sides see is partial, in the sense of incomplete and in the sense of skewed in a direction that feels right. I am also suggesting that what we see—what we think is the fact of the matter—is intimately related to how we think we ought to act. The orientation to the world that feels right affects what we see, and what we see affects how we think we ought to act.[i] I broached this issue concerning the two sides' different conceptions of what *is* and how we *ought* to act in the preceding chapter, when I observed the connection between the two sides' "anthropologies" and their "ethics"—between what they think the nature of human beings is and what they think our ethical responsibilities are. In this chapter I explore how each side's conceptions of what technology is, what human nature is, and what nature is are interrelated—and I also explore how each side's conceptions of what those things are is "entangled"[2] with its conception of how we ought to act.

DEFINITIONS AREN'T
EPISTEMOLOGICAL GUARDRAILS

When we engage in academic debate, however, it is to our strategic advantage to overlook the entanglement of our conception of what is (the facts) and our conception of what ought to be (our values). One way to overlook these entanglements and to support our ethical conclusion is to speak as if we proceeded to our conclusion

---

i One of many additional sorts of "entanglement" is that how we act not only reflects but also affects what we see and feel.

from definitions of one or more of the debate's key terms—to speak as if we used reason alone to discover those definitions.

We speak as if, once we have given clear definitions of key terms like *technology* or *nature* or *human nature*—once we have said what each of those things is—we will have secured the basis for the right answer to some hard ethical question. We sometimes seem to hope that the right definition, which reflects the true nature of whatever is being defined, can serve as a sort of epistemological guardrail, which will keep us on the ethical road. Indeed, the hope that the right definition—the right understanding of the nature of something—can give us guidance about what we ought to do, may be a secular version of the hope that God or Nature will provide such guidance.[ii]

The abortion debate is one of the easiest places to see how high our hopes can run for the right definition. People who oppose abortion sometimes hope that once they've defined a person as a being with human DNA, they will have demonstrated that abortion is wrong. Presumably, reasonable observers just need to supply the noncontroversial premise that killing persons is wrong. People who support abortion rights, on the other hand, sometimes hope that once we've defined a person as a being with, for example, self-awareness, we will have shown reasonable observers that abortion can be right. Presumably, reasonable people just need to supply the noncontroversial premise that killing *non*persons can

---

ii In the terms of the previous chapter, when we reify a concept like *person* or *authenticity*, we hope we have discovered a solid foundation from which we announce our equally solid ethical conclusion, as in "See, abortion is wrong!" or "See, medicating children is right!" As I will suggest in the next chapter, we have to resist reifying personhood and authenticity *and* we need to engage in ongoing conversation about what those terms mean. Making decisions requires that we use definitions and requires that we remember that, contrary to our fondest hopes, those definitions aren't epistemological guardrails.

be right. Bluntly: both sides can build their ethical conclusions about abortion into their definition of persons.

I should clarify that, when I say both sides build their conclusions about technologically shaping our selves into their definitions, I don't mean to suggest that this process is deliberate. My guess is that it usually isn't. Moreover, I don't mean to suggest that the influence between conclusion and definition goes just one way. I suspect that we also bring to the debate definitions of key terms that both look right from our stance toward the world and that make us more likely to reach one conclusion rather than another. The arrows of influence, as it were, go both ways: the conclusion that looks and feels right lines up with the definition that looks and feels right. Whichever way the arrow goes at any given time, more than reason alone is at work in the definitions we use and the conclusions we pronounce.

The problem isn't that we build our conclusions into our definitions. Those conclusions (and the definitions we use to defend them) often entail deep insights. The problem is forgetting that we do this building in. As we will see, in the context of the debates about technologically shaping our selves, the problem is that we still sometimes seem to imagine that our definition of technology, our specification of what it *is*, can provide disinterested support for our view of whether we *ought* to use some new technology.

FOR CRITICS, TECHNOLOGY IS "UNNATURAL" OR "ARTIFICIAL" AND ITS VALENCE TENDS TO BE NEGATIVE

For critics of emerging technologies, technology is by definition what comes after human beings come on the scene, and nature is what was there before them. On such a view, human beings use technology to breach nature. Technology is "artificial," or, as critics sometimes lapse into saying, it is "unnatural."[3]

And, at other times, critics speak as if technology is what is, by definition, "not social," when they distinguish between *technological* and *social* means of achieving some desirable end. An example of this is to suggest that, whereas medication is a technological means for promoting psychological health, counseling is a social means. The implicit assumption is that, to the extent that our means are "social," they are not technological, and to the extent that they are not technological, they are not unnatural and thus are more likely to be good. A negative valence is there from the beginning, both in the critics' definition of technology as unnatural (or artificial) and in their distinction between technological and social means.

Where does the negative valence associated with technology come from? Surely not just one place. I speculate, though, that at least in part it is, as a geneticist trying to explain the emergence of some complex human trait might say, "associated with" what we might call the critics' "tragic" conception of human nature. According to that conception, human beings' greatest assets are always inextricably linked up with, if not the same as, their greatest defects. Here, most simply, the human capacity to use technology to improve our selves is the very same capacity as the one that gives us the power to harm them. On such a view, it is inevitable that we will inadvertently produce harm while in the noble pursuit of improvement. The critic worries about the inadvertently but harmful results of our actions, which she thinks are an inevitable result of our nature as human beings. I take the negative valence associated with technology to be a trace of that conception of human nature.

It isn't hard to see some resonance between the critics' "tragic" conception of human nature and the "ecological" lens, which, in the previous chapter, I suggested they bring to their analysis of efforts to technologically shape our selves. Critics worry that, in the context of the fragile ecosystems that are our bodies and societies, our noble efforts to improve one of our capacities will inadvertently but inevitably harm another. We try to fix one problem and in the process create another, often worse one. Think here of the worry that, if we were to engineer out the sort of depression that afflicted Abraham Lincoln, we might inadvertently engineer out the empathy and wisdom that enabled him to meet his country's greatest moral challenge.

In the gratitude stance, some lenses are more likely than others to seem apt—whether the lens through which technology is artificial, or the lens through which human nature is tragically flawed, or the one through which nature is a fragile web. From the gratitude stance and through lenses such as the ones I just mentioned, some ethical conclusions are far more likely than others. Because I find the gratitude stance and the cluster of lenses that we often use when we adopt it to be valuable, I would like others to do the same. But I also want to remember the partiality of my stance and lenses. I want to remember that they help me see some things and make it hard if not impossible to see others. Critics have not looked out into nature and disinterestedly discovered what technology is. Nor has God told them what it is. Nor did the interpretive skills they learned in school give them access to the right definitions. Their stance and lenses are useful, particular, and partial.

FOR ENTHUSIASTS, TECHNOLOGY IS "NATURAL" AND ITS VALENCE CAN BE POSITIVE

It is perhaps harder to see at first, but the enthusiasts, too, can build an awful lot into their conception of what technology is. Below

I will describe how, from the creativity stance, technology looks to be value-free or morally neutral. Now, however, I want to say how, from the creativity stance, technology looks to have a straightforwardly positive valence. For the enthusiasts, technology is not unnatural but, on the contrary, is the most natural thing in the world. As the authors of the first presidential-level commission on the bioethics of genetic engineering wrote in a 1982 report, *Splicing Life*, nature itself has long been a genetic engineer: after all, bacteria have forever spliced viral DNA into bacterial genomes.[4] Or as Robert Carlson, who is enthusiastic about newer forms of genetic engineering, observes, nature has built power factories forever: once upon a time primitive forms of large cells incorporated into themselves smaller cells to serve as power sources. Carlson has in mind how, for example, animal cells today include power generators called mitochondria, just as plant cells today include power factories called chloroplasts. As Carlson puts it, "Biology is technology. Biology is the *oldest* technology" (emphasis in original).[5] Nothing could be more natural than technology. Animal cells use it. Plant cells use it. Even bacterial cells do.

To see another way in which enthusiasts build a positive valence into their understanding of what technology is, it helps to compare their and the critics' understanding of the relationship between "technological" and "social" means. As I mentioned above, critics tend to define technology by distinguishing between technological means and social means and also by assuming that social means entail a sort of self-evident goodness that technological means don't. Enthusiasts (at least in the technologically shaping selves debates) accept that same assumption regarding the goodness of social means, when they define technology such that "technological" means are identified with—not distinguished from—the means that the critics would call "social." This is what enthusiasts are getting at when they speak, for example, of education as a technology for learning.[6,iii]

Moreover, according to the enthusiasts, even if we could distinguish between technological and social means of altering the world and our selves, we wouldn't have learned anything about why we shouldn't use a given technology. There's nothing more natural, or more in keeping with human nature, than humans using technology.

Where does the positive valence associated with enthusiasts' conception of technology come from? At the risk of appearing to impose more symmetry than could possibly be there, I would suggest that if there's a way in which the critics' intuition regarding human nature and the world is tragic, there's a way in which the enthusiasts' intuition is "comic" in the ancient sense of comedy: a vision of the world where all of the parts that seemed to be at war in the beginning are in the end harmonized into a happy whole. That is, the enthusiasts fully recognize the potential problems associated with the technological interventions at hand but are sanguine about our ability to resolve them.

And it isn't hard to see some resonance between that comic, sanguine conception of the human predicament and the "engineering" lens I alluded to in the previous chapter. On the enthusiasts' view, no matter how huge are the problems we create, we can engineer our way out of them. When the hopes for human genetic

---

iii Students of Foucault will notice that his conception of "technologies of the self" is much closer to the enthusiasts' understanding of what technology is than it is to the critics' understanding. For Foucault, a nun's disciplining of her body by means of prayer and fasting is as much a technology of the self as is the actor's disciplining of his body with surgery and pharmacology. See Michel Foucault, *The History of Sexuality, Volume 1*, trans. Robert Hurley (New York: Vintage, 1978), and *Technologies of the Self: A Seminar with Michel Foucault*, ed. Luther H. Martin, Huck Gutman, and Patrick H Hutton (Amherst: University of Massachusetts Press, 1988). On the other hand, Foucault's understanding of normalization and medicalization is much more in keeping with the critics' worry than with the enthusiasts' hope.

engineering first began gaining currency in the 1980s, some enthusiasts averred that such engineering might be humanity's only
hope of adapting to the environment that we have, with our exu-
berant use of our technologies, despoiled; we might, for example,
genetically engineer ourselves to survive in an atmosphere con-
taining less oxygen than our current one.[7] More recently, others
have argued that there is a moral imperative to do research on
Mars, on the grounds that, once we have made our current planet
uninhabitable, we will need another.[8] That is, the enthusiasts' cluster of lenses—including their understandings of what technology
is, what nature is, and what human nature is—enables them to
articulate a stance toward the world, from which no challenge
can't be met with another, newer, better technology.

Whereas the critics tend to think of human vices and virtues as
inextricably linked, the enthusiasts are hopeful about our capacity
to unlink them. The enthusiasts are, as I mentioned in the preceding chapter, hopeful about the modularity of our virtues and vices,
even about our ability to engineer in the virtues and engineer out
the vices. They are deeply sanguine about our capacity to, as the
boilerplate has it, embrace the promise and avoid the peril. So, like
the critics, the enthusiasts come to these debates from somewhere
in particular. And also, like the critics, the enthusiasts build their
ethical conclusions into their definitions of key terms like technology, nature, and human nature.

SLIPPING FROM IS TO OUGHT

Another way of putting this point about how we build our ethical
conclusions into our definitions is to say that we slip between
claims about what technology *is* to claims about whether we *ought*

to use it. Even those who pride themselves in resisting the urge to make what David Hume called the "imperceptible change" between what is the case to how things ought to be find themselves making that change.[9]

Because I think those prone to enthusiasm will be especially dubious about my claim that they, too, slip imperceptibly from facts (or definitions) to values (or ethical conclusions), I want to develop that claim. Specifically, I want to consider in more detail how the enthusiasts' putatively factual observation concerning what technology is changes imperceptibly into their ethical claim that technology is either good—or, as we will see, that it is "morally neutral."

Toward the end of the last century, Donna Haraway was one of the most prominent articulators of the idea that it is the nature of human beings to alter our selves. According to Haraway, it is time to see our selves for what we have been all along: cyborgs.[10] On her account, there is nothing more natural than the merging of human beings and technology; indeed, it makes utterly no sense to try to parse the technological and the natural (or the technological and the social). Again, on the enthusiasts' account, the technological *is* natural. Or as the philosopher Andy Clark puts it, human beings are "natural-born cyborgs."[11]

To better understand what Clark means when he says that we are always already fusions of "natural bodies" and "technologies"—and thus how he, too, represents the technology-is-natural view—it helps to consider briefly an essay he published with David Chalmers called "The Extended Mind."[12] Perhaps the easiest way to understand Clark and Chalmers's claim that "our minds already extend beyond our skin bags" is to consider an example they give, which I will paraphrase.

Imagine two people, each of whom is wandering around midtown Manhattan. Each decides to go to the Museum of Modern Art (MoMA). The first person, Inga, is a middle-aged woman with a healthy brain. What does she have to do after it occurs to her that she wants to go to MoMA? She has to remember its address. On Clark and Chalmers's account, Inga has to, as it were, pull up MoMA's address from the part of her brain, her hippocampus, where memories are stored. Once she has retrieved the information from the so-called repository in her brain, she can start walking in the right direction.

The second person is Otto. It also occurs to him to go to MoMA, but he is elderly and suffers from memory loss. Fortunately, he carries around in his pocket a handwritten list, which contains the addresses of his favorite places. Otto reaches into his pocket, pulls out the list, "remembers" where MoMA is located, and starts walking.

Clark and Chalmers know that many of us assume there is an obvious and significant difference between the means that Inga uses to remember (her hippocampus) and the means that Otto uses (the paper with the writing on it). Inga's means of remembering is located inside her "skin bag" and Otto's means of remembering is located outside of his. Some might ask, What could be more significant than the boundary between what's inside and outside of our body?

But it is precisely the assumption regarding the significance of that boundary that Clark and Chalmers reject. They sum up their extended mind hypothesis: "If, as we confront some task, a part of the world functions as a process which, *were it done in the head,* we would have no hesitation in recognizing as part of the cognitive process, then that part of the world *is* ... part of the cognitive process" (emphasis in original).[13] They believe that only prejudice makes us think that Inga's memory is part of her mind but that Otto's writing isn't part of his. Insofar as Inga and Otto both perform the same cognitive task of retrieving information, Otto's piece of paper with the list on it is as much a part of his mind as Inga's hippocampus is part of hers. On the Clark-Chalmers view, it is arbitrary to distinguish between means of remembering that are within the skin bag and those outside it.

As I understand their argument, Clark and Chalmers are not speaking metaphorically. They intend the extended mind hypothesis to give an account of the world as it is, and they are exhorting us to get over the prejudice that there is something ethically significant about the line drawn by our "skin bags." On their view, empirical investigation reveals that our minds extend beyond our skin bags. They are saying that, *by definition*, any technologies we think with, from writing and books to drugs and computers, are part of our minds.

The philosopher Neil Levy has made explicit what he takes to be the ethical implications of that factual claim about the way our minds are.[14] He argues that, if we recognize that our minds are always already extended by technologies like writing and computers, we should grant the ethical parity between efforts to enhance cognition with technologies like those which intervene directly inside the skin bag, and efforts to enhance cognition with social means, which intervene indirectly, from outside it. That is, if we see clearly what mind *is*, we will see that there is no prima facie reason to think that an "indirect" method of changing someone's mind with, for example, education is ethically preferable to a "direct" method of changing someone's mind with, for example, medication. The critics' distinction between technological and social means, Levy suggests, is ethically arbitrary.

And as I mentioned in the preceding chapter, Levy is perfectly explicit about the particular understanding of the nature of human beings that he brings to his analysis of using new technologies to shape ourselves: we are by nature creative animals. New technologies help us do what we do naturally. We might say that, to allay the critics' worry about the unnaturalness of technology, Levy observes the respect in which it is perfectly natural.

Levy's conclusion is deeply important. My point is simply that it reflects partial understandings of what mind, human nature, nature, and technology *are*—and that, ultimately, it reflects a stance toward the world and our selves that is partial. Partiality isn't bad, it's inevitable. What can be bad, though, is succumbing to the temptation to forget the partiality of our views.

TECHNOLOGY AS VALUE-*FREE*

In summing up his argument that it is irrational to suggest that a given human intervention is bad because it is "unnatural," John Stuart Mill wrote, "*All* human action whatever consists in altering, and all useful action in improving, the spontaneous course of nature" (emphasis added).[15] Mill's first point here is that, insofar as all human action consists in altering the course of nature, it is irrational to worry that any one action alters its course. It's a bit like worrying that birds use their wings to alter currents of air. Mill's second point is that, instead of worrying about whether a given intervention changes the course of nature, we should worry about whether that change is "useful" for human beings.

In other words, according to the enthusiasts, technologies themselves are value-free or morally neutral. Through this lens, insofar as technologies can be put to good or bad purposes, they aren't inherently good or bad. As enthusiasts reasonably point out, murderers use knives, but so do surgeons. Muggers use guns, but so do hunters trying to feed their families. Terrorists use airplanes, but so do humanitarian aid workers. On this account, human beings have values, technologies don't.

So for the enthusiasts, if there is something to worry about in the context of technologically shaping selves, it doesn't have to do with any technology in itself but with the purposes to which humans put it. Notice that, at this moment in the debate, the enthusiast is using the lens through which technology is a morally neutral means, together with the lens through which persons are free subjects. As I mentioned in chapter 2, when I introduced the metaphor of binocularity (and as I will discuss at length in chapter 6), the enthusiast emphasizes—at this moment in the debate—the respect in which we are subjects who can freely choose the ends to which we put technology. The enthusiasts are sanguine enough about human nature to believe that, over the long haul, we will choose good purposes over bad ones. It is difficult to exaggerate the importance of the enthusiasts' insight regarding the respect in which technologies are morally neutral and the respect in which human beings have the capacity to choose between good and bad uses of them.

TECHNOLOGY AS VALUE-*LADEN*

Critics of enhancement, however, have a different insight regarding the nature of technology. According to them, technology is not a morally neutral or value-free tool but is a value-laden frame.[16] In this way, or at this moment in the debate, critics tend to emphasize the respect in which human beings are objects, shaped by social, political, and historical forces beneath or beyond our ken. Moreover, critics emphasize that those forces infiltrate or become expressed in our technologies. Critics think their job is to uncover the values, which are always embedded in technologies and which escape the attention of the casual observer. On the critic's view, the enthusiast is naïve in her estimation of the extent to which we are free and our technologies are value-neutral. On the critic's view, technologies shape, or frame, our experience, but that influence is as hard to see as gravity. The philosopher James Edwards puts the critics' point succinctly when he writes, "Technology is a frame that blinds us to itself as a frame. It is a way of revealing [the world to us] that makes us forget that it is *a* way of revealing."[17]

A simple example can begin to illustrate the critics' point. To detect the presence of genetic abnormalities such as the one associated with Down syndrome, physicians now offer prenatal testing technologies to all pregnant women in the United States. In principle, this technology can be used either to prepare for the birth of a child with Down syndrome or to selectively abort a fetus with such an abnormality. No one holds a gun to women's heads to make them choose either way, so there is a respect in which it is fair to say that women freely choose to use the technology for one purpose or the other: they can use the technology to selectively abort an affected fetus or they can use it to prepare for a child with a disability.

As the critic reminds us, however, it is also true that this technology has shaped the pregnancy experience and choices of many women and their partners. Since the introduction of prenatal genetic testing, the birth of children with Down syndrome is so rare in some social groups that it is assumed that *the* purpose of the technology is to identify and selectively abort fetuses carrying the Down trait. In this demographic, if prospective parents don't use the technology, and bring a child with Down syndrome into the world, they risk enduring the opprobrium of their peers.[18] "How could you be so ignorant as not to have known about this technology? Or if you did know about it, why didn't you use it?" That is, the fact that a technology exists can swiftly, if imperceptibly, turn into an ethical obligation to use it for a specific purpose.[19]

Critics take prenatal genetic testing to exemplify the capacity of a technology to shape us; it shapes our understanding of how prospective parents should act. Specifically, it shapes our experience of pregnancy and our experience of the pregnancy of others. In that sense, the technology isn't morally neutral or value-free but is value-laden. Moreover, it is laden with values of a particular sort, the sort that people with Down syndrome don't embody: like efficiency, speed, and success in the marketplace.

Critics don't worry only that the technology-is-morally-neutral view ignores the fundamental respect in which we are objects shaped by technological and other forces beyond or beneath our awareness. They also worry that our technological way of being in the world will turn us into objects in a different sense: the more our technologies proliferate, the more we will be tempted to treat each other as if we were "mere objects," not human. They worry that, if we don't check our technological imperative,[20] we will become dehumanized.[21] Critics worry that, if we look at the natural world ever more as a "standing reserve," as a source of "raw material for us to manipulate and exploit to advance our comfort," we will ever more look at other human beings and even ourselves in the very same ways.[22]

INSIGHT AND OBFUSCATION

While the critics are good at seeing how our technologies are value-laden, they tend to be bad at recognizing the respect in which we ourselves are always already laden with technology. That failure of recognition may be a cost associated with the critics' insight. (Like Milton Friedman's lunches, insights are never free.)

To clarify this point that enthusiasts reasonably suggest critics are prone to forget, it helps to begin with the simple fact that our earliest ancestors had much larger guts, and much smaller brains, than we do. Before the invention of tools for cooking, our ancestors ate raw foods. Because extracting sufficient metabolic energy from uncooked foods required that they eat relatively enormous amounts, they needed guts much larger than the ones we have today. According to "the expensive tissue hypothesis," for our brains to increase in size, without a concomitant increase in the size of our overall budget of metabolic energy, our guts had to decrease in size.[23] For that to happen, our predecessors had to become more efficient at absorbing nutrients, which is what new technologies enabled them to do. Our brain-based ability to use new technologies to exploit the energy from what we ingested— both by cooking foods and by acquiring energy-richer sources such as nuts—made it possible for our guts to decrease in size, which presumably in turn made it possible for our brains to expand still more. With still larger brains, our ancestors created more elaborate technologies, which continued to reshape our brains and ways of being in the world.

Accounts like that move enthusiasts to emphasize that, insofar as Homo sapiens are always already shaped by technology, there's nothing ethically new about new technologies. We've been doing it all along: inventing technologies, which shape every facet of our bodies and our environments, and thus ultimately shape our selves. In that way, it is perfectly reasonable to say that we are always already laden with our technologies.

Insofar as the enthusiasts' account is correct, the critics have to recognize that the distinction between our "original" natures and our "technologically shaped" natures is far less sturdy than they seem to wish. That original nature, which presumably preceded our use of technology, isn't as unchanging as we like to imagine when we appeal to it as a sort of epistemological guardrail, much less moral guidepost. There is an important respect in which critics are just wrong when they speak as if, "out there" independent of or prior to us, there is a standard—unadulterated human nature—against which we can measure our interventions and somehow infer what we ought to do.[24]

Of course, the critics aren't the only ones whose insights come at a conceptual cost. To begin to see one of the biggest costs associated with the enthusiasts' skepticism about making distinctions between nature, human beings, and technology, it helps to recall the criticism heaped on the government-appointed administrator of the BP Deepwater Horizon Disaster Victim Compensation Fund, Kenneth Feinberg, when he said of the catastrophic oil spill in the Gulf of Mexico, "I think this is a natural spill, a natural disaster."[25] He and the others who repeated his claim were interpreted to be trying to insinuate that it was nature, not the human beings who ran BP, that was responsible for the devastation wrought by the explosion of the rig.[26] As I have already indicated, if that is what he was insinuating, there is a sense in which it is a sophisticated claim. There's a sense in which the distinctions between nature and human beings and human technology are arbitrary, and thus a sense in which the explosion was indeed wholly "natural."

The obvious and considerable cost of the enthusiasts' rejection of distinctions like the one between nature and human beings, or between human beings and human technologies, however, is that they give up one way of talking about the special role that human beings play in the world. They give up one way of talking about the special place that human beings occupy in nature—in virtue of our remarkable, natural capacity to use tools to transform it. Jettisoning those distinctions altogether leaves us with one fewer way of criticizing developments that threaten some features of our lives that are good, like clean oceans. Jettisoning those distinctions altogether can be as ethically unhelpful as imagining that articulating the right definitions will save us from going off the ethical road.

If there is an important sense in which critics suffer from what some enthusiasts have called a "status quo bias" against new technologies,[27] there is also a sense in which the enthusiasts suffer from their own variety of "status quo bias": they tend to be biased in favor of accepting more of the same, where ever-expanding technological intervention into our selves and the rest of the natural world is the status quo.[28] Choosing wisely in the future will require resisting both varieties of status quo bias.

A MORE BINOCULAR APPROACH TO TECHNOLOGY

Earlier in this chapter, I acknowledged that when I first came to the debates about technologically shaping our selves, I spent a lot of energy trying to establish that means matter morally—in the hope that establishing that would be a reason to resist at least some technological interventions. New technological means seemed, and to some extent still do seem, to be integral to a status quo that I often find alienating. Insofar as new technologies can be especially good at expressing values like efficiency, speed, and control, arguing against those technologies was for me a proxy for arguing against those values. It was a way of arguing for the values that, by nature and nurture, I find congenial (for example, engagement, slowness, and letting things be). While I certainly have not given up the insight that technologies are laden with values, I have had to give up any notion that it is useful to speak of a given technology as if it were inherently problematic. I have had to accept the usefulness of oscillating between the insight that technology is value-laden and the insight that it is value-free. I've come to adopt a more binocular habit of thinking about technology, where I don't have to choose between the insight that it shapes our ends and the insight that we use it to pursue our ends.

So, I suggest, technologies can frame our experiences in ways that make us feel increasingly alienated and stressed out, and we can use technologies to facilitate our efforts to engage in the sorts of activities that can be essential constituents of our flourishing. As the great critical commentator on technology Albert Borgmann allows, though our "technological culture" can alienate us from the sorts of "focal practices" that make animals like us truly happy, they can also "call forth engagement."[29] Making music together depends on the technologies that produce instruments, sharing meals together depends on our technologies for food preparation, walking long distances at older and older ages depends on technologies that protect our feet. As the philosopher Maartje Schermer might put it, these technologies do not "disrupt," but rather "amplify," focal engagement.[30] As we will see in the next chapter, we should not rule out the possibility that, in spite of all of the potential dangers, a technology like a drug might also facilitate our ability to engage in the world as we take it and our selves truly to be.

As I now look back on my initial foray, many years ago, into the enhancement debates, I can see the way in which my desire to talk about how means matter was partly a function of my desire, as a secular, pluralist liberal, to avoid the appearance of talking about ends. After all, like John Stuart Mill, I am eager to respect individuals' conceptions of their own "experiments of living,"[31] and I am loath to interfere. Perhaps like the repressed, however, talk about ends always returns: we are the animals who ask, How ought we to live? What ought we to do? What ends or purposes should we pursue? So in the next chapter I will, finally, broach the question concerning the ends to which we should put our technological interventions.

Chapter 5

Nobody's against True Enhancement

I have been suggesting that when our desire to win an argument allies with the binaries that undergird our languages, we can end up making conceptual choices that are plainly at odds with our desire for understanding. No thoughtful person would want to choose between thinking that technology is value-free and thinking it is value-laden. No thoughtful person would want to choose between thinking that we are by nature creators or creatures, or that nature is a mechanism or a web. She would not want to choose between saying that reason, power, and control are important features of our being or that emotion, vulnerability, and mutuality are. She also would not want to say that we should accept all suffering or that we should attempt to extirpate it all. Nor would she want to choose between saying that (as I have already mentioned and will discuss at length in the next chapter) human choices are free or determined. Yet, when we—critics and enthusiasts alike—enter into arguments, we can speak as if we believed that intellectual clarity and courage required us to make such choices. The views we articulate in public debate can thus become far more "monocular" than the understanding we desire.

I also suggested that the critics and enthusiasts about enhancement in particular and technological intervention in general share a fundamental moral ideal, which they tend to forget they share in the heat of academic combat: the moral ideal of authenticity, according to which we owe it to ourselves to be true to ourselves. They share the ideal of us identifying and striving toward worthy goals, which are not imposed on us by any outside party, such as the church or state, but are truly ours. They agree that it is our job to find our own way of being happy, or flourishing.[i]

In this chapter, I want to further pursue my suggestion that the two sides of the debates about technologically shaping our selves share more than their rhetoric sometimes seems to indicate. I want to emphasize the extent to which critics and enthusiasts share the notion that human flourishing consists in engaging in activities in the world, as the world, and as we our selves really are. I will suggest that if we got better at noticing that shared understanding, it would be easier to go from arguing for or against enhancement to having a conversation about what real or true or, yes, "authentic" as opposed to "false" (or merely putative) enhancement is. We could go from arguing for or against technological intervention to having a conversation about whether a given intervention will promote or thwart someone's flourishing, where each of us is understood as an individual, whose right to flourish in her own way has to be protected against the community, and who, as a member of a community, has an obligation to consider the impact of her projects on others.[ii]

---

i I take "happiness" and "flourishing" to be equally decent translations of Aristotle's term *eudaimonia* (*Nicomachean Ethics*, Book I). They are both names for what human beings want—not for the sake of something else (in the way we want, say, money), but for the sake of itself.

ii As friends of the extended-mind hypothesis might put it, the more we understand the respect in which our minds extend beyond our skin bags, the less we can rest easy with the principle that the only way you really can harm me is by bloodying my nose. On the extended-mind view, "I" extend way beyond my nose.

NOBODY'S FOR SOMA

When critics argue against enhancement, they often invoke the specter of Soma, the drug in Aldous Huxley's *Brave New World* that allowed people to take a holiday from the world as it is, to enjoy ongoing intoxication, without any of the usual nasty side effects. Critics worry that, ultimately, the enthusiasts' enthusiasm will lead to a world where human beings are satisfied by a pill, in the absence of engaging in the sorts of activities that normally produce a sense of happiness or flourishing.

I have not, however, been able to find a single enthusiast who is enthusiastic about Soma. Not one. James Hughes, who in *Citizen Cyborg* is as enthusiastic as anyone, explicitly rejects the prospect of a drug that would give us a permanent feeling of intoxication and would keep us from pursuing the sorts of goals that human beings normally pursue. He writes,

> Imagine...we [develop a drug that] is 100% and permanently addictive. The drug might rewrite the brain so that all goals and values become secondary to remaining intoxicated. *Suppressing or discouraging such a drug* would be an exercise of coercion *in the defense of liberty*, keeping people from selling themselves into slavery [emphasis added].[1]

Those prone to criticism and those prone to enthusiasm agree: a drug like Soma would enslave us. It wouldn't liberate us to do what we want most: to engage in activities in the world as it is. It is important to keep in mind that both sides would refuse Soma, not because it is an enhancement but because it is not a "true" enhancement. It wouldn't promote anyone's flourishing.

Robert Nozick's famous philosophical thought experiment can help us better understand the common ground that critics of and enthusiasts about enhancement share. In it, Nozick invites us to imagine that we can hook ourselves up to an "experience machine."[2] This machine would allow us to enjoy all of the sensations that normally grow out of engaging in activities, but without actually having to engage in them. If you normally seek the pleasurable feelings associated with reading, or running, or feeding the hungry, or healing the sick, or playing music, or making love, or making trades on Wall Street, the machine could give you those feelings directly, and you wouldn't have to go to the trouble of engaging in those activities. If you normally seek difficult or even painful sensations, the machine could give you those, too. You could have whatever mix of feelings you usually enjoy—without having to engage in the activities that usually give rise to them. The experience machine would stimulate your brain to simulate the identical sensations.

Nozick was not inquiring about whether we would like to take a temporary break from the usual relationship between our actions and feelings. He understood how much we desire such breaks, and as far as I know he never argued against wine. Nor was Nozick inquiring about whether we might experience regret upon unhooking from the machine. He stipulates that the hookup would be permanent.

So, would you choose to hook yourself up to a machine that gave you exactly the internal feelings or experience that you normally have when you engage in activities in the world? One logically possible, and to Nozick's mind disingenuous, answer is: "Look, if the internal feeling or experience were *exactly* the same, then it is arbitrary to prefer the old-fashioned sort to the simulated sort. Maybe I wouldn't be playing a guitar, but, per the condition of the experiment, I would feel exactly the same as if I were. Maybe I wouldn't be engaged in an intimate conversation, but I would feel exactly the same satisfaction as if I were." According to this skeptical rejoinder to Nozick's question, the preference for engaging in activities in the world as it is and as we are is mere prejudice.[3]

I would suggest that, if the preference for engaging in activities in the world as it is and as we are is a prejudice, it is a prejudice in the way that our preference for sociality is. Most human beings appear to share this desire for contact with the world as it is, and this is about as fundamental a fact about our selves as we're likely to find. No matter how wonderful the feelings produced by the experience machine might be, and no matter how wonderful it would be to escape the difficulties that can arise when embodied beings engage in activities in the world, we don't seem to want the feelings without really engaging in the activities that produce them. As Jonathan Glover succinctly puts it, "We want to do things, not just passively receive experiences."[4] To lend support to my assertion that you, too, share that desire, I want to begin by considering one example that is exceedingly bound by time and culture: thinking about love can help us notice that we, too, want to engage in activities in the world, as it really is and as we really are.

A PILL TO CREATE LOVE

In *Beyond Therapy* the President's Council on Bioethics (PCB) offers a scenario that makes a deeply important point. They invite us to imagine a young man at a party who is under the influence of the drug Ecstasy and who begins a conversation with a woman he has never met before. He tells her that he loves her and wants to marry her. The PCB invites us to imagine that the man means what he says "insofar as the feeling he now has is indistinguishable from what he might one day feel when he truly falls in love with a woman." That is, the drug produces a perfect simulation of the feeling he might one day have while under the influence of a flesh-and-blood human being. Then the council asks, "Should the fact that this man's feelings are produced by the drug, rather than inspired by the woman, matter?"[5]

The PCB concludes, rightly I think, that it should matter to the woman and to the man. It should matter to her because she wants to be seen as she truly is, not as the drug makes her seem. And it should matter to him, insofar as he should want his love to be real. As the council puts it, "The young man's drug induced 'love' is not just incomplete—an emotion unconnected with knowledge of and care for the beloved. It is also unfounded, not based on any-thing—not even visible beauty—from which such emotions nor-mally grow."[6] On the PCB's account, neither the man nor woman should want a love that has essentially been created by the drug alone.

Even we who fancy ourselves to be post-postmodernists—we who are skeptical of reification and Truth—are here thrown back on some version of binaries like true and false, real and apparent, authentic and inauthentic. Even as we remember the respect in which such binaries are obstacles to our understanding, we remember the respect in which they are essential for it. Without them, we can't think or speak about the sort of love we want for ourselves and for those we love (such as our children).

We want to be loved for who we truly are. We wouldn't, for example, want to be loved by someone who was ignorant of our defects or mistaken about our gifts. We want to love others as they truly are, too; we wouldn't want to love someone who only appears to be loveable. We would be distraught to discover, for example, that the partner we thought was a fine writer was in fact a plagiarist. And we want others' love for us—and ours for them—to be true; we would be crushed to learn, just before we died, our partner had only pretended to love us for all those years. Moreover, we want our feelings of love to grow out of engaging in activities with the person we love. We don't want to settle for the feelings produced by a drug alone, any more than we want to settle for the feelings simulated by Nozick's experience machine.

Perhaps you are asking, Who is "we"? Certainly not everyone who ever lived or even who lives today. Again, romantic love is a recent and culture-bound invention. I am, however, suggesting that "we" does include critics *and* enthusiasts engaged in the debates about technologically shaping our selves. Lest you think that "we" refers to critics only, or even more narrowly, only to critics who find the PCB's language congenial, notice that even someone as prone to enthusiasm about technologically shaping our selves as John Harris agrees with the council about the "pill for love." He says explicitly that the PCB is right: "We don't want a pill to make us feel that our lover loves us—we want to be loved."[7]

And Harris is by no means alone among those prone to enthusiasm in objecting to a "pill for love." Julian Savulescu and Anders Sandberg define a good marital relationship as "one which both parties desire and which gives each pleasure, and allows or facilitates each to lead lives which are objectively valuable."[8] To advance their argument, Savulescu and Sandberg make a useful distinction, which reveals an important value commitment they share with their academic foes, the President's Council. They distinguish between using a drug to *maintain* a loving relationship and using a drug to *create* such a relationship. Specifically, they endorse using technology to maintain a relationship that is founded on shared perceptions of the goodness of the other and on sharing experiences that grow out of such perceptions, but they reject using technology to create the feelings normally associated with such perceptions and experiences. As Savulescu and Sandberg put it, "The use of drugs to instill a new love is more likely to create inauthentic love, since the causal reasons for the love may lie in the drug . . . rather than the particular person loved." It is, on their view, acceptable to use a drug to maintain a loving relationship, but not to create one out of a drug alone.

That is, neither critics nor enthusiasts want to create love out of whole cloth, in the absence of the feelings and experiences normally associated with it. I suggest that the critics' and enthusiasts' shared rejection of a "pill for love" has everything to do with their shared commitment to the value of us engaging in activities in the world, as we really are, as others are, and as the world really is. They reject it because, to use John Harris's apt phrase, the pill "would constitute no sort of enhancement."[9] It's a putative or fake—not a true—enhancement. The enthusiast's commitment to creatively transforming our selves has limits, and, as we are about to see, the critic's commitment to letting our selves be does, too.

A PILL TO MAINTAIN LOVE

Whereas Savulescu and Sandberg object to an imaginary pill that would create love out of whole cloth, they say that marriage counseling is a perfectly fine way to maintain a love relationship. It's hard to imagine that the President's Council would object to marriage counseling, if it aimed at facilitating, for example, the sorts of intimate conversation that maintaining a love relationship requires. One might nonetheless ask, Given the PCB's explicit concerns about drugs as a threat to authenticity, would they go along with the enthusiasts in endorsing *a drug* that facilitated the sort of talk that can help to maintain a relationship? (Such a drug is not merely hypothetical; Ecstasy has apparently been used by some marriage counselors for the purpose of facilitating talk-based counseling, and some have suggested that the hormone oxytocin might be used for the same purpose.)[10]

In fact, the President's Council does not object in principle to the use of drugs to help us pursue "true happiness." They are explicitly open to the value of using drugs, if such use facilitates true human flourishing. The PCB writes:

> Would the pharmacological management of our mental lives draw us toward or estrange us from the true happiness that we seek? It is hard to answer in the abstract. *In some cases, it might bring us nearer, by restoring our natural ability to take satisfaction in joyous events and satisfying deeds.* In other cases, it might estrange us, by substituting the mere feelings divorced from their natural and proper ground [emphasis added].[11]

That is, the PCB, which is famous for its concerns about the uses to which such drugs might be put, is also open to the possibility that drugs might in fact "draw us toward" the forms of engagement with others and the world that we desire. They are eager to warn us of the danger of alienation, but they acknowledge the possibility that such drugs could promote our flourishing, our authentic engagement with the world as it is. At least in principle, we have reason to believe that the council would be open to a drug that would facilitate the ability to engage in the sorts of conversations that are necessary for "maintaining" a loving relationship.

You might ask, however, Is the PCB nearly *as* "open" as enthusiasts like Savulescu and Sandberg? The short answer is no. At one point, Savulescu and Sandberg imagine a scenario that would surely appall members of the PCB. They invite their readers to imagine a woman who takes herself to be in a good and loving relationship with a man who happens to be prone to promiscuity. They also invite their readers to imagine that, in an effort to maintain her relationship with him, this woman might freely choose to take a drug that allows her to tolerate her husband's promiscuity.

Actually, it strikes me that, for Savulescu and Sandberg to be consistent, they, too, should reject the promiscuity-toleration pill on the same grounds they rejected a pill that created the feelings of love out of whole cloth. In both cases, rather than facilitating engagement with the world as it really is, the pill distances the wife and husband from it. That is, endorsing the promiscuity-toleration pill seems to violate one of Savulescu and Sandberg's own deepest commitments.

Am I trying to suggest that there are no substantive differences between critics like the President's Council and enthusiasts like Savulescu and Sandberg, that they really think the same thing? That would be absurd. They come to these debates from different stances and emphasize different insights, which are easiest to see through the lenses that are most congenial to them. As a pluralist, I want to affirm the reality of differences. That is, I want to notice and embrace the reality of the moral worth of different stances.

At the same time, however, I suggest that, in the heat of academic battle, we can overstate the magnitude of those differences. Both enthusiasts and critics would refuse a pill that created the feelings of love out of whole cloth, because the two sides share a fundamental commitment to us being in contact with the world as it is, as we are, and as others are. And both sides should endorse a pill that would help facilitate or maintain a loving relationship, insofar as it would help us pursue that commitment: to gain a deeper relationship with the world and others as they are. Next, more briefly, I want to suggest another context in which we can see that the substantive differences between enthusiasts and critics aren't as great as their rhetoric sometimes suggests.

BATTLING OVER MEMORY

In that same volume about enhancement that contains the discussion about a pill for love, the President's Council on Bioethics (PCB) initiated a conversation about the ethics of using drugs to blunt the intensity of emotions associated with painful memories.

Before getting to their view concerning such memory drugs, however, I should first make a more general comment regarding the PCB's stance. Enthusiasts have grown accustomed to assuming that critics (such as the authors of the PCB report) want to *ban* what Allen Buchanan has called "the enhancement enterprise."[12] Such an assumption doesn't come from nowhere. Some of the critics' rhetoric is surely to blame. But it's important to recognize the extent to which that assumption misconstrues the critics' considered position.

It is, for example, hard to square the enthusiasts' charge that critics want to "ban" enhancement in general with Francis Fukuyama's explicit and highly developed call for regulation. Yes, in *Our Posthuman Future*, Fukuyama does say that cloning should be "banned outright, for reasons both intrinsic and tactical"[13] (as did Leon Kass in "The Wisdom of Repugnance"[14] and as Jürgen Habermas seems open to in *The Future of Human Nature*[15]). However, Fukuyama also says that what we need in general is a "more nuanced regulatory approach." Specifically, he says that "a totally laissez-faire attitude toward biotech development, *and* the attempt *to ban* wide swaths of future technology—*are misguided and unrealistic*" (emphasis added).[16] Indeed, at the very end of *Beyond Therapy*, the PCB itself says that it has "sought to begin [to understand the enhancement enterprise], in the hope that these first steps might spark and inform public debate, so that *however the nation proceeds, it will do so with its eyes wide open*" (emphasis added).[17] That is not exactly a clarion call for an across-the-board ban on "the enhancement enterprise."

Though, as I just mentioned, the PCB didn't offer a single policy recommendation about any technological intervention—unless we count the recommendation that the nation proceed "with its eyes wide open"—the volume's often portentous tone, with its mention of evildoers and its allusion to Lotus eaters, elicited portentous responses. In one of them, specifically concerning memory blunting, three coauthors, in the *American Journal of Bioethics* (AJOB), floated the possibility that the PCB might be advocating that the state become the "enforcer" of "a religious fundamentalism that claims divine knowledge of right and wrong."[18] They added, "If this were not the PCB's intent, it surely would have reassured the reader to the contrary." Once again, though, I think some rhetoric on both sides obfuscates some fundamental points about which critics and enthusiasts agree.

MEMORY ERASURE

We in the West have long contemplated what it would mean to not only blunt the emotional intensity of some memories, but also erase them altogether. Homer sang of Odysseus's visit to a land whose inhabitants ate mythical Lotus flowers, which made humans forget everything they ever knew. Upon eating the mythical flowers, several of Odysseus's men completely forgot their earlier lives. They became blissfully contented, as Tennyson much later would retell it, to "lie reclined on the hills like Gods together, careless of mankind." The erasure of Odysseus's men's memories made them inhuman.

Insofar as erasing all of our memories would be tantamount to annihilating our selves,[19] a drug for total memory erasure would separate us from the world as it is and from our selves as we really are. Though the coauthors of the piece in AJOB that I mentioned above—whom I refer to here as "the AJOB authors"—did not address the theoretical possibility of total memory erasure, they do allow that "memory and its relationship to emotion clearly are vital to human functioning and flourishing and are very complex."[20] That is, it seems fair to infer that, like the criticism-prone PCB, the enthusiasm-prone AJOB authors would also be against eating Lotus flowers.

THE CASE OF LADY MACBETH'S MEMORY

As we saw earlier, the PCB thinks that for us to truly flourish, or to be truly happy, we need to engage in meaningful activities and be with others. On the PCB's view, we don't just want the feeling of happiness or flourishing or fulfillment that working well or loving well normally produces. We want to engage in the activities that normally give rise to those feelings. Moreover, we want to engage with the world as it truly is. Or, as they put the same point in the context of their discussion of memory, we don't want to "separate the subjective experience of memory from the truth of the experience that is remembered."[21]

To help us grasp what they mean when they speak of the importance of maintaining a connection between what we feel and how the world really is, they invite us to think about Macbeth's request that his doctor free his wife from the painful memory of her murderous scheming. The PCB suggests it would be bad if Lady Macbeth could take a pill that eliminated her pangs of conscience. After all, the magnitude of her guilt was proportionate to the monstrosity of her acts. To sever the link between her acts and her proportionate experience of guilt would be to commit a fundamental ethical mistake. If a human being didn't feel suffocating guilt after committing such acts, the world would be "out of joint."

If we consider the AJOB authors' treatment of the "medicalization" of memory, we can see why they should, in principle, share the PCB's concern about giving Lady Macbeth a drug that eliminated the suffering that attends her painful memories. The term *medicalization* comes from sociology, and it names the process by which we increasingly conceive of "normal human problems" as medical problems.[22] The tacit assumption is that it is a mistake to use medicine or technology to eliminate some problems that are normal for human animals: as in, it is normal to feel guilt when one has unjustly harmed another, or to feel anxiety in anticipation of battle, or to feel grief when one's partner dies. (I will have more to say about the term *normal* in chapter 7.)

The AJOB authors invite us to imagine a future in which a pharmaceutical company creates an advertisement for a drug like propranolol, which is already being used in attempts to reduce the sting of painful memories associated with Post-Traumatic Stress Disorder (PTSD). In this hypothetical ad, however, the company suggests that the drug could be used by someone "after an embarrassing or humiliating experience at the office." The AJOB authors worry about such a scenario. As they put it, "Here we have reason to be concerned that a private company seeking to sell more pills will promote an expansive set of PTSD causes and symptoms (to physicians and patients alike), altering both our sense of the illness and our interpretations of the experiences that might cause it."[23] They don't, and they don't need to, say why they are concerned with "altering our sense of the illness and our interpretations of the experiences that might cause it." They can rightly assume that their readers share the assumption that it is a fundamental mistake to sever the act of humiliation and the suffering normally associated with being humiliated. If a human being didn't suffer upon being humiliated, the world would, again, be out of joint.

The enthusiasm-prone AJOB authors' example of the office worker who would take a pill to reduce the normal emotional distress associated with the normal experience of embarrassment or humiliation is not as evocative as the criticism-prone PCB's example of Lady Macbeth taking a pill to reduce the guilt and emotional distress that normally accompanies treachery. It's also true that, whereas the humiliated office worker's stress is in response to a wrong that was done to him, Lady Macbeth's distress is in response to wrongs she did. What's important to notice, however, is that both groups agree that we should seek to distinguish between normal human suffering that is proportionate to some normal human experience, and suffering that is not.

The two groups agree that we should learn from the experiences that produced those painful emotions—or perhaps we should exit or change the situation or behavior that produced them. They agree that at least some sorts of suffering should be tolerated rather than blunted or erased. This doesn't make them masochists or sadists. It makes them willing to accept that, while some forms of suffering can poison our lives, others can be a source of growth. Indeed, there is an expanding literature that finds that posttraumatic *growth* is not only real but also more common in the wake of traumatic events than is PTSD.[24] At any rate, we can see the respect in which the AJOB and PCB authors agree that it would be bad to take a drug that alienated us from our true experience of how we and the world truly are—every bit as much as we can agree that notions like "alienation" and "true experience" are essentially contestable.

TREATING PTSD

The AJOB and PCB authors don't agree about just the badness of eating Lotus flowers and the badness of reducing Lady Macbeth's anguish. That is, they don't only agree about both the badness of erasing memories, which would deprive us of having identities at all, and the badness of a drug that would blunt emotions that are painful but normal, or proportionate to some true fact about the world. They also agree about the goodness of using drugs to blunt the emotional sting of memories, when the intensity of those memories is *dis*proportionate to what triggers them and is incapacitating—as in the case of PTSD.

If one did not experience profound distress in the wake of participating in a war, something would be amiss. But that is not the experience to which PTSD refers. The person with PTSD experiences anxiety in civilian settings that is disproportionate to the events that trigger it. Intense anxiety might be a proportionate and lifesaving response to seeing a bump in the road on the battlefield in Afghanistan, but it would be a disproportionate and incapacitating response in a parking lot in New Jersey. Refusing to treat the veteran's PTSD would be wholly inconsistent with the PCB authors' commitment to promoting the conditions that allow humans to truly flourish. As the PCB authors acknowledge, the traumatic memories associated with PTSD can "cast a shadow over one's whole life, making the pursuit of happiness impossible."[25]

As I suggested earlier, neither the PCB members nor the AJOB authors want to, as the PCB put it, "interfere with the normal psychic work and adaptive value of emotionally charged memories."[26] The two groups agree that intervention is appropriate, if it facilitates growth. This facilitation can take different forms, which both sides endorse, even if the PCB's tone reveals a deep wariness of pharmacological means. The PCB credits a neuroscientist with saying that drugs (like propranolol) "might make it easier for trauma survivors to face and incorporate traumatic recollections, and in that sense could facilitate long-term adaptation." Such drugs might, for example, provide a physiological foundation upon which trauma survivors can engage in psychotherapeutic activities. Ever more evidence suggests that some forms of psychotherapy do for PTSD sufferers precisely what the PCB—and, presumably, AJOB authors—would want: to facilitate the sorts of learning and growth that constitute, and make possible, what both sides would recognize as human flourishing.[27]

Just as earlier we saw the enthusiasts and critics agree that we should not create love out of whole cloth with a pill but should be willing to use a pill to facilitate the sorts of activities that make real love possible, so here the enthusiasts and critics agree that we should not obliterate painful memories with a pill but should be willing to use a pill to facilitate the sorts of remembering that make living well possible. Neither side wants a pill that gives a feeling of happiness in the absence of activity, or that precludes activity.

Furthermore, both sides would endorse a pill that makes it possible to engage in precisely the sorts of activities (therapeutic and otherwise) that, as Peter Kramer put it long ago, open us up to human tragedy and, as we might put it, true human happiness or flourishing.

CONCLUSION

If reasonable people agree about the goodness of intervening when it facilitates our ability to engage in the sorts of activities that produce true happiness, and if they also agree about the badness of eating Lotus flowers or reducing Lady Macbeth's (or the humiliated office worker's) anguish on the grounds that such interventions would separate us from ourselves and the world as they really are, does this mean that critics and enthusiasts don't ever really disagree? Of course not. There is an inevitable zone of ambiguity between those interventions that critics and enthusiasts can agree would be bad because they sought to erase a proportionate response to the world as it is, and those interventions they can agree would be good because they would facilitate someone's ability to engage in the world as it is.

As I have suggested, people coming to the technologically shaping selves debates from the creativity and gratitude stances tend to emphasize different, but equally salient, features of human beings. Those prone to emphasize creativity will have a rather more expansive conception of the range of cases in which we should intervene, and those prone to emphasize gratitude will have a less expansive conception. There surely will be cases in that zone of ambiguity, where reasonable people will reach different but equally decent conclusions. The line between proportionate and disproportionate responses to experience isn't any brighter than any other line in ethics.

We can respect those different conclusions and also remember what critics and enthusiasts share, which I take to be even more fundamental: a commitment to helping people to avoid interventions that would cut them off from the world and themselves as they really are, and to promote interventions that promote their ability to engage with the world as it is and as they are.

If my interpretation is reasonable, critics *and* enthusiasts would reject Soma, a pill for love, Lotus flowers, and a pill for the eradication of all painful memories. They wouldn't reject those interventions because they are enhancements, however, but because they are not. Those are all examples of "putative enhancements"— interventions that promise to make us happier or to flourish more fully but that really would separate us from the necessary condition for true human happiness or flourishing: being in contact with the world as it is and as we are.

I have been suggesting that if we are to get better at discussing the questions concerning technologically shaping our selves, we need to get over indulging the pleasure we can take in being *for* or *against*. We need to get over our tendency to suffer from what Freud called the narcissism of small differences.[28] The harder, more fruitful task, which I have gestured toward in this chapter, is to talk together *about* what true enhancement or improvement is and *about* whether a given intervention will promote or thwart it.

If we are to have that more fruitful conversation, we need to get better at resisting the sort of monocular thinking that moves us to speak as if technology is value-free or value-laden; as if nature is a mechanism we can engineer or a fragile web we should let be; as if human beings are by nature creators or creatures. We need an approach that is better at remembering that such binaries are both necessary for, and obstacles to, exploring the questions that matter most to us. Remembering that would conduce to a more binocular habit of thinking.

Ultimately, though, I want to say something about how we can get from a binocular approach to thinking to a binocular approach to acting. In particular, I suggest (in chapter 7) what a binocular habit of thinking *and* acting might look like in the clinic, when families have to make decisions about whether to use surgery to try to normalize the appearance of their children. To prepare the ground for my articulation of a binocular process in the clinic, however, I need first to return to the subject and object lenses I first discussed when, in chapter 2, I introduced the metaphor of binocularity. That is, before attempting to say something about how we should respect persons in the clinic, first I want to say more about what persons are. I want to make the case for getting over the monocular approach to understanding persons, which can seem ever more seductive as the natural sciences teach us ever more details regarding the fact that we are objects. I want to say more about a binocular approach, which is equally good at noticing the fact that we are objects and the fact that we are subjects.

Chapter 6

Comprehending Persons
as Subjects and as Objects

In this chapter I want to explore how seeing our selves as subjects *and* as objects can help us understand our selves in greater depth than, as we are wont to do, seeing our selves as subjects *or* objects. I want to suggest the value of comprehending our selves as beings with minds, who can (to differing degrees) have the experience of being free, and as objects, which are not free but determined by an infinite number of forces—including genes, neurons, hormones, microbiota, nutrients, desires, reasons, customs, institutions, geography, and history. I'm after a way of comprehending our selves that takes seriously the experience of what it is like to be a subject[1] and takes seriously the myriad, infinitely complex mechanisms that are the necessary condition for that experience. To perceive human beings in depth, we need to try to understand what it is like for someone to be herself, just as surely as we need to try to explain the forces that give rise to that experience. We need the first-person and third-person perspectives—or, in my lingo, the subject and object lenses. Few things are easier, though, than succumbing to the temptation to consider our selves through only one.

AN OLD FORM OF MONOCULARITY

There is a long intellectual tradition in the West that emphasizes a conception of human beings[i] that is commonly called "dualistic." (I say "emphasizes" because, no thinker—much less tradition—is as simple as we make it sound when we seek to make a point.) Dualistic conceptions, which can be traced at least to Plato but which come to most of us today by way of Christianity, hold that persons are constituted by two parts or two kinds of substance. One part, often called soul or mind, is eternal and really real. It is not a physical or (as Descartes would say) "extended" thing, so it is not affected by the same laws as the rest of the things in the natural world. That first part, which can't be affected by "mere" natural forces, is, on such dualist accounts, the seat of our freedom. The second part, the body, on the other hand, is impermanent and illusory. At best, the body is a vessel for or temple of the soul; at worst, it is "no more than" an obstacle to choosing freely.

Requesting your patience for a moment, I want to suggest the way in which such a *dualistic* understanding is *monocular*. Again, with the term *monocularity*, I am referring to what happens when we succumb to our proneness to conserve mental energy, and we content ourselves with the one lens (or one cluster of lenses) that feels most congenial. According to what I'm calling monocular accounts of human beings, only one of the two lenses *really* counts. On the sort of Christian understanding I'm referring to here, it is the mind (or soul) that is salient and that makes freedom

---

i I will use the terms *person* and *human being* interchangeably. I don't hope to add anything to the debate between those who want to expand the circle of beings that count morally in the direction of embryos and those who want to expand it in the direction of dolphins.

possible. On such an account, only one of the two parts that constitute persons—the mind—is taken to be real. Indeed, the sta-
bility, reality, and truth of the mind or soul are established in
comparison with the impermanence, unreality, and illusoriness
of the other part, the body. The unreality of the body, as it were,
shores up the reality of the mind.

I should reiterate that my objection to the sort of dualist
account of persons that I'm describing here is surely not that it
takes the mind or "subject lens" seriously. I am deeply eager to
take seriously our experience of being subjects, of having intentions and purposes. Rather, my primary objection is that such an
account takes *only* the subject lens seriously. It assumes that, to
understand what persons are, we don't really need to consider
them as objects. On such an account, the body is "no more than"
what distracts us from, or obstructs our view of, the really
real: the soul or mind. The body is in an important sense
"epi-phenomenal": it is below or beyond, and secondary in significance to, the really real phenomenon, which is the mind. This
sort of dualism is monocular insofar as the subject lens alone is
taken to be sufficient for understanding what's really real about
human beings.

A CONTEMPORARY FORM
OF MONOCULARITY

Strange as it may sound at first, some, though, of course, not all,
contemporary neuroscientific thinking can succumb to a different version of the same mistake that I just attributed to Christian
dualism. That is, some neuroscientists engage in their own form
of monocularity. In the ardency of their passion to reject what

I've referred to as Christian dualism, some neuroscientists end up with what we might think of as Christian dualism on its head. The new account of persons entails the same two parts as did the old account, but it just flips the valuations of those parts. On such a neuroscientific account, it is the brain (or body) that is the really real, and it is the mind (or soul) that is illusory or epi-phenomenal. Insofar as such an account suggests that the experience of being a subject is an illusion, and that all we really need to consider is the way in which we are objects, such an account is monocular.

Such monocularity can be glimpsed in a book, *Portraits of the Mind*, compiled by the neuroscientist Carl Schoonover.[2] Though "mind" is featured in the title, the book itself offers a history of brain science in gorgeous pictures, beginning with a second-century C.E. drawing of the optic nerve and ending with beautiful contemporary representations of activity in the visual cortex that are constructed from fMRI data. In the first paragraph of the book's foreword, the neuroscientist and popular science writer (who has since gone in for heavy criticism for matters unrelated to the following point) Jonah Lehrer says,

> The first time I saw a naked cortex, freshly removed from its bony encasing, I was struck by its bloodiness. There was no soul here, just a thinking machine made of flesh....I couldn't believe that I had emerged from a similar mass, just these three pounds of meat with the texture of Jell-O.[3]

After saying that he finds it easy to sympathize with those who over the ages have thought that we needed "something else," something nonphysical to explain our experience, Lehrer delivers the bad news: "And yet, there is nothing else: this is all we are." Or, as the neuroscientist Joy Hirsch puts it in the last essay of the book, "mind *is* brain" (emphasis added).[4]

This contemporary form of monocularity—where mind is reduced to brain, where what's really real is the brain, and where, for all intents and purposes, the mind is epi-phenomenal and can be jettisoned—is hardly unique to Hirsch, Lehrer, and Schoonover. As we are about to see, it is exceptionally easy to slip from the observation that we don't need any extranatural or metaphysical stuff to explain the emergence of mind, to the claim that mind *is* brain, and to speak as if mind is an illusion.

A CLOSER LOOK AT THIS CONTEMPORARY FORM OF MONOCULARITY

Francis Crick, a codiscoverer of the structure of DNA, turned to neuroscience later in his career. Specifically, he sought to understand human consciousness, to isolate what he called the "neural correlate of consciousness." He wanted to explain what goes on in the brain that is correlated with, and presumably gives rise to, the experience of being conscious. Discovering the neural correlate of consciousness would presumably entail solving the perennial problem of how our experience of mind or consciousness emerges out of physical matter.

In 1994 Crick published *The Astonishing Hypothesis.*[5] (Crick acknowledges in that book his large debt to Christof Koch, who published his own elaboration of their hypothesis ten years later, in *The Quest for Consciousness.*)[6] In *The Astonishing Hypothesis,* Crick distilled into plain language a conception of mind that persists in the neuroscience literature today, a conception that I am calling "monocular." In the book's introduction, Crick states his astonishing and now-famous[ii] hypothesis: "'You,' your joys and your sorrows, your memories and your ambitions, your sense of personal identity and free will, are in fact no more than the behavior of a vast assembly of nerve cells and their associated molecules."[7] Please notice the scare quotes around *you*. "You" think that you are something special, the bearer of joys and sorrows, memories, ambitions, a sense of identity, and a free will. But that's an illusion. "You" are really "no more than" a vast assembly of nerve cells.[8]

Crick sets out his view in explicit opposition to Christian dualism. In particular, he articulates it in opposition to the conception of soul and body found in the Catholic catechism, which he quotes in order to reject: "The soul is a living being *without a body*, having reason and free will" (emphasis added). Contrary to Christian dualism, according to which we need some immaterial, extranatural, God-given stuff to explain how we have consciousness, Crick breaks the news that no such stuff exists.

For those like Crick—and for me—it is, indeed, important to recognize that we do not need any extranatural or metaphysical stuff to explain the emergence of mind, soul, consciousness, subjectivity, or freedom. I am eager to grant that, in that sense, it is completely, absolutely true that we are "no more than" a vast assembly of nerve cells.

But in his passion to say that mind, understood as something composed of immaterial or extranatural stuff, is an illusion, he speaks as if mind is an illusion, full stop. He slips from reasonably assuming that the emergence of mind can (in principle) be

---

ii His formulation is now so famous that it is used in psychological experiments aimed at exploring how beliefs about free will affect moral behaviors. See, e.g., Kathleen D. Vohs and Jonathan W. Schooler, "The Value of Believing in Free Will: Encouraging a Belief in Determinism Increases Cheating," *Psychological Science* 19, no. 1 (2008): 49–54.

explained in terms of material, to unreasonably assuming that such an explanation makes talk of mind obsolete. In the throes of his enthusiasm, he slips into speaking as if we should just jettison silly, folksy talk about mind. We should just stop talking about, for example, "you" being free. While Crick himself didn't seem prepared to follow his thought quite that far, some neuroscientists and neurophilosophers have, with claims that personhood and freedom are illusions—perhaps very valuable illusions, but illusions nonetheless.[9]

Although Crick believes that one day we will be able to elucidate how neurons give rise to consciousness altogether, he readily acknowledges that we aren't close to being able to do that today. So, in *The Astonishing Hypothesis*, he adopts the more modest goal of elucidating how neurons give rise to *visual* consciousness, to vision. He believes that if he can show that seeing "is all done by the neurons," and not by any soul or mind or subject, he will have shown why we should stop speaking as if mind were more than brain. We will, he believes, have no choice but to accept that mind *is* brain.

Please do not be confused by the fact that, whereas I am using the metaphor of binocularity to name my approach to thinking about the nature of persons as objects and subjects, Crick is using the science of vision to establish his principle that, to understand persons, it will suffice to use the object lens—the lens that considers us solely as bodies or, even more narrowly, as brains.

CRICK'S ARGUMENT FOR JETTISONING "YOU"

Crick adopts a two-pronged strategy to show that we don't need anything other than neurons to explain visual consciousness and that, by extension, we don't need anything more than brain to explain consciousness or mind or subjectivity altogether. In the first prong, Crick rehearses what neuroscientists know about the mechanisms that make vision possible. And what they know is truly remarkable. He explains what is known at the level of neuroanatomy: how, for example, information in the form of light is processed by the retina, which, by means of chemical and electrical changes, is then transmitted along the optic nerve, which branches, thus sending information through different specialized areas of the brain, which is then transmitted farther along to, and then up and down, the hierarchically organized visual cortex. He also explains what is known at the level of the anatomy of individual neurons, which, again, is remarkable: that, for example, some neurons in the visual cortex respond selectively to only particular features of the visual field, such as the disparity between lines or the orientation of objects in space.

Crick adduces such anatomical and physiological details to support his view that we don't need "more than" neurons to explain vision any more than we need "more than" brain to explain mind. As I have already said, there is a sense in which I think that's exactly right: we don't need any extranatural stuff to explain mind. My objection becomes clearer in considering the second prong of Crick's strategy.

If the first prong is to show what neuroscientists do know about vision, the second is to show what you don't know about vision. Specifically, it's to show that you don't know what you see the way you think you do. As he succinctly puts it, "What you see is not what is *really* there; it is what your brain *believes* is there" (emphasis in original).[10] Crick invokes a couple of sorts of evidence to support his assertion, the first of which involves a different sort of appeal to neuroanatomy. He begins by urging us to consider more carefully what we think we see when we look out into the world.

Specifically, he urges us to reconsider our assumption that we see a continuous picture of the world.

If I stretch out my right arm and lift my index finger to about the level of my nose, I can, of course, see it. It seems to occupy what looks to me like one part of a continuous picture of the world. But if I move my arm, say, toward my right, a point will come (when my arm is at about a 45-degree angle to my torso) where I can no longer see my finger. Then, if I keep moving my arm still farther to the right, my finger comes back into view. We call that part of the visual field where I can't perceive my finger "the blind spot." I can't perceive my finger there because that part of my visual field corresponds to the place in my retina where there are no neurons that can process visual information. The cells in that part of my retina constitute my optic nerve, which exits my retina, headed to my visual cortex. So, Crick suggests, a basic fact of neuroanatomy allows us to grasp that, though I think I see a continuous picture, I don't really. It's an illusion.

A second sort of evidence that Crick invokes entails another kind of optical illusion. In this kind, we think we see one thing but really see another. Our mind plays a trick on us, much as the magician does when he makes us think we watch him saw his shapely assistant in half as she lies in a box on a gurney.[11]

Imagine an abstract painting in a rectangular frame, with its long sides oriented in the horizontal direction. And imagine that the background of the picture starts out dark on the left but becomes gradually lighter toward the right side of the frame. Imagine that we then place a horizontal band of *uniform* (dark) color across the middle of the picture. Even though I know that the band really is of uniform darkness, it will look to me like the band becomes lighter as the background becomes darker. But again, it's an illusion. I think I see a band that is lighter on the left side of the picture and darker on the right, but I don't.

But if what I think I see isn't what I really see, where does the picture I think I see come from? According to Crick, it can come from only one place: the brain. The brain is the complex mechanism that takes fragmentary, discontinuous information about the world and, as it were, creates a re-presentation of the world. I don't see the world as it is; I see it as my brain makes it seem.

On such an account, the brain is acted on by incoming information or stimuli, which the brain processes to create a picture. Such an account has no need of, or patience with, the concept of mind, at least insofar as that concept entails taking someone's experience of seeing seriously. On such an account, the subjective experience of seeing (or of having an intention or purpose or aim) is epi-phenomenal; it is "no more than" a by-product of the incoming stimuli.

In that way Crickian accounts of mind are monocular: they suggest that the object lens alone suffices to give an account of visual consciousness and, ultimately, of consciousness altogether. Please notice that I do not call such an account monocular because it uses the object lens. I call it monocular because it uses *only* the object lens, because it imagines that it has explained away the need for the subject lens.

SOCIAL SCIENTISTS, HUMANISTS, AND MONOCULARITY

I want to emphasize, however, that neuroscientists are hardly the only ones tempted to use only the object lens. To see how we in the humanities and social sciences engage in our own form of monocularity, it helps to consider the strategy that so many of us use when we interpret human behavior, engaging in what the philosopher Paul Ricoeur called a "hermeneutics of suspicion."[12]

Traditionally, *hermeneutics* referred to strategies of interpreting texts. When Ricoeur coined the phrase "hermeneutics of suspicion," however, he was referring to a strategy of interpreting human behaviors, in particular, a strategy that adopted a suspicious attitude toward subjective experience. In practicing a hermeneutics of suspicion, one looks beneath the manifest, illusory surface of human behaviors to understand the latent reality going on below. In the case of the three great hermeneuts of suspicion whom Ricoeur invokes—Marx, Nietzsche, and Freud—what one sees beneath the surface for them, respectively, is money or power or sex.

While Crick wants to understand our selves in terms of neurons, not money or power or sex, like all hermeneuts of suspicion, he wants to uncover what's really going on beneath the surface. If we look beneath the surface of our conscious, "subjective" experience, hermeneuts of suspicion agree, we glimpse the forces that do "the real" work—whether neurons or genes or capital or power or sex—and that give rise to the less real, manifest subjective experience. According to the hermeneuts of suspicion, we are constituted by forces we aren't conscious of, and to truly comprehend our selves, we need to focus first of all on precisely those forces. (In the next chapter we will see how useful this lens can be, if it isn't our only lens.)

Also like those older hermeneuts of suspicion, Crick hated organized religion, insofar as it professes knowledge of mind (or soul) that is made of extranatural or metaphysical stuff. And, as I mentioned above, according to traditional religions, perhaps especially the Christianity that Crick grew up around, mysterious, extranatural stuff was invoked to explain the reality of our subjective experience, in particular, the reality of our experience of free choice.

As I, too, am steeped in the hermeneutics of suspicion, I also am committed to rejecting any religious account of human subjectivity that appeals to extranatural stuff. However, I also want to remember the world-transforming profundity of those religions at their best: when they offer an empirical observation regarding the nature of human subjectivity and offer an ethical interpretation of that observation. The empirical observation is that each of us is a site of subjective experience, and that for each of us, our own subjectivity is infinitely valuable. At their best, organized religions have taught us, against the grain of our all-too-natural tendency to imagine otherwise, that as a matter of fact other human beings value their subjective experience as much as we value ours and that we ought to respect their valuation of their experience as we would have them value ours.

What these religions have said we share, and what they have exhorted us to respect in each other, cannot be glimpsed through the object lens. That's just not what it's for. The object lens isn't for understanding the felt experience, or "subjectivity," of human beings. The third-person perspective of the sciences—looking through the object lens—may someday give a complete *explanation* of how subjective experience arises in animals like us. But, by definition, it can't give us *understanding* of the first-person perspective. The third-person perspective can't give us understanding of what it is like for a particular human being to be the site of experience. It can't by itself give a full account of human beings, and thus it doesn't give a reason to, as Crick suggested, jettison talk of "you."

To understand what it is like for a particular human being to be her, we have to ask her and then listen to her reply. To assume we know what it is like, just because we know the mechanisms that give rise to that experience, is at best naïve and at worst dangerous. To take seriously this real feature of animals like us—our subjectivity—requires that we recognize the need for what I've been calling "the subject lens."

Again, when you and I talk about mind or soul, we don't need to invoke the sort of immaterial, extranatural stuff that the authors of the catechism did. We don't need to believe that "the soul is a living being without a body, having reason and free will." We can reject those authors' explanations of how our experience arises, while affirming their efforts to take seriously our experience of having free will or of having purposes and making plans to achieve them. Similarly, we can reject the tendency of Crick and the hermeneuts of suspicion to think of that experience as illusory, while affirming their effort to explain how that experience arises. Our aspiration should be to get better at oscillating between the object lens, which is for explaining how our experience arises, and the subject lens, which is for understanding what it is like to have such experience.

INTERLUDE: TWO TRADITIONS OF THINKING ABOUT THE AIMS OF NATURAL SCIENCE

Secular, pluralistic liberals like I am have a tendency to imagine that our conception of the natural world is, well, natural—in the sense of its being unsullied by any particular value commitments. We have a tendency to think that there is nothing particular about our conception of nature or our attitude toward it. Just look at the universal language of mathematics that modern natural science depends on. The science that Chinese or Indian or Nigerian researchers do isn't in principle any different from the science done by American or British researchers. They all submit their work to the same journals, abide by the expert decisions of the same judges, and so on. Indeed, the modern, natural scientific view is so pervasive that it doesn't seem like a particular view at all.

But the modern, natural scientific view entails very particular philosophical and value commitments, which are easy to glimpse when we compare this view to, for example, ancient natural science. For an ancient natural scientist like Aristotle—just as for today's modern natural scientists—it was important to try to explain how things work. Aristotle, too, was deeply interested in the mechanisms that make organismal life possible. But different from modern natural scientists, Aristotle thought that studying living organisms scientifically also required attending to their "purposiveness" or "aim-directedness." On the ancient account, the natural scientist seeks to take seriously not only how we work, but also why. He seeks to understand us as mechanisms and also as "more than" mechanisms: as subjects or agents.

Unfortunately for those of us committed to the moral equality of all human beings, Aristotle did not speak only about the "purposiveness" of human beings; he didn't speak only about the fact that we have intentions and pursue purposes. He also spoke about what he took to be *the* purpose of human beings. On his account, the purpose or end of human beings is to engage in virtuous activity in accordance with reason. I said "unfortunately" because purpose in that sense was part of a larger hierarchical way of understanding the structure of nature, which helped him to justify slavery. That is, for Aristotle, some human beings were by nature capable of engaging in the sorts of virtuous activity in accordance with reason that would be a true fulfillment of human nature, whereas other human beings were not. With such an understanding, if some human beings are by nature suited for virtuous activity in accordance with reason, and others are not, then some human beings are fit to rule and others to be ruled. Some humans are, by nature, fit to be philosophers and others to be slaves.

We can face up to that deeply ugly feature of Aristotle's philosophical biology, while also appreciating what was deeply beautiful about it: he sought to take seriously, as a natural scientist, the fundamental fact that organisms intend or desire to pursue some ends and to avoid others. That is, Aristotle took seriously what so many modern natural scientists bracket as "epi-phenomenal": the intentions and purposes we have vis-à-vis the world.

Whereas that ancient tradition of natural science aspired to *see* (or "contemplate") organisms, to understand them in their wholeness, in their pursuit of purposes, and in their distinctive ways of being in the world, modern natural science, which is often traced to Francis Bacon or Rene Descartes,[13] aspired to *see through* those alleged purposes to what was really going on. (To this extent, Bacon and Descartes were "hermeneuts of suspicion" long before Marx, Nietzsche, and Freud.) By seeing what was really going on beneath the surface, by understanding the mechanisms that gave rise to the appearance of purposiveness, the modern natural scientists sought to master and transform the natural world and the organisms that inhabited it. Specifically, they aimed to transform human beings and their world to relieve human beings of the suffering that so often plagued them. Eventually, Bacon hoped, modern natural science would not only rid human beings of disease, but enable them to live forever. Medicine as a means to immortality is hardly the invention of the transhumanists.

Any of us who has ever taken an antibiotic, or vaccine, or pain-killer can appreciate the spectacular success of the modern, natural scientific effort to understand the mechanisms that constitute us and to, in light of that understanding, transform us. My point is to remind us of the way in which, for all of its power and universality, modern natural science reflects a particular conception of what nature really is, as well as what our attitude toward it ought to be. Mastering nature (as embraced by modern natural science) and contemplating nature (as embraced by ancient natural science) are surely not mutually exclusive attitudes, but each is value-laden and particular.

USING THE SUBJECT LENS

The ancient, natural scientific attitude never completely disap-peared from the West, though it was, beginning in the 17th cen-tury, eclipsed by the rise of the modern natural scientific attitude. While that eclipse continues today, there was in the 20th century an effort to revive the ancient aspiration to take seriously the human experience of having aims and purposes. That effort, undertaken in very different ways by philosophers such as Edmund Husserl, Martin Heidegger, Maurice Merleau-Ponty, and Hans Jonas, is often referred to as "philosophical phenome-nology." Those 20th-century thinkers did not seek to *see through* the purposes of organisms to understand what mechanisms gave rise to them; rather, they sought to (using my lingo, not theirs) *see* those purposes as they are experienced by individual subjects.

Alva Noë, to whom I owe my attention to Crick, is part of that phenomenological tradition, which seeks to understand human beings as creatures enmeshed in a world, who have desires, purposes, and intentions vis-à-vis that world.[14] As for Aristotle, for Noë subjectivity is an essential feature of being human. It isn't an epi-phenomenon. On the contrary, to understand the reality of being human, we have to investigate what it is like to be in the world and to have purposes vis-à-vis it. We need to take seriously "the subject lens."

Above I suggested that, for Crick, consciousness is what happens when the brain processes incoming information from the world, and out of that information creates a representation of the world in our brains; in this sense, on Crick's model, the brain is a creator. As an antidote to Crick, Noë offers what we might (hearkening back to chapter 3) call an "ecological" account of consciousness or mind. For Noë, consciousness is what happens when, as he puts it, creatures are enmeshed in, and intentionally oriented to, a world.[iii] The reason that, in spite of my blind spots, I experience a continuous picture of the world is that I am always already in the world, constantly adjusting to and interacting with it. When I say I see, I'm not talking about something that can be understood *adequately* by referring to what's happening in my brain, within my skull, though, of course, I couldn't have the experience of seeing at a given moment if what's going on in my brain at that moment weren't going on.

When I say I see, I refer to my experience of being in the world. To suggest, as Crick does, that what I see is my brain's creation is, according to Noë, to miss a fundamental feature of being a

---

iii In chapter 3 I observed that enthusiasts tend to emphasize that we are by nature creators and that critics tend to emphasize that we are by nature creatures. You would not be wrong to notice an analogous terminological situation here, where enthusiasts tend to emphasize that our brains are "creators" of representations of the world and critics tend to emphasize that we are "creatures" who have access to the world as it is. In both cases, I see the apparently competing lenses to offer valuable insights.

creature like me: the experience of being in the midst of something I have not created but that is there nonetheless and that I have developed the skills to access, millisecond by millisecond. I don't experience a blind spot in my visual field because I am constantly adjusting to, gaining access to, those features of the world that interest me. According to Noë, we will not adequately understand seeing if we conceive of it as my brain taking (and then filling in the missing bits of) a picture:

> What I see is never the content of a mental snap shot; the world does not seem to be reproduced inside of me. Rather—and this is the key—the world seems available to me. What guarantees its availability is, first of all, its actually being here, and second, my possessing the skills needed to gain access to it.[15]

To be fair, Crick says explicitly that he does not want to say (even if he sometimes sounds like he's saying) that vision is like a series of snapshots of the world taken and developed by the brain. But Crick does want to say that seeing is all done by the neurons. He does want to say that what we think we see isn't what we really see, that what we think we see is a representation of the world created by our brains.

Noë, on the other hand, urges us to think that, most of the time—he is aware of optical illusions and magic tricks—what we think we see is what we really see. For Noë, a key to grasping the inadequacy of the view that visual consciousness is created by the brain is to recognize the sense in which we are, as he puts it, "out of our heads." On his view, visual consciousness does not happen within our skulls. It is not something we create, but rather something that happens to creatures enmeshed in, and purposively oriented to, a world. He urges us to think of consciousness less as a thing created by our brains and more as a way of being oriented toward the world. Noë writes:

> The world is not a construction of the brain, nor is it a product of our own conscious efforts. It is there for us; we are here in it. The conscious mind is not inside us; it is, it would be better to say, a kind of attunement to the world, an achieved integration.[16]

For Noë, our experience of being in the world, and having purposes vis-à-vis it, is not epi-phenomenal. The subject lens is essential for comprehending what sorts of animals we are.

To insist that we need to use the subject lens to comprehend persons in depth is not to diminish the need for using the object lens. We are subjects in the sense that we have experiences that demand understanding, and we are objects in the sense that those experiences admit of explanation. To comprehend persons in depth, we need both lenses.

FROM THINKING TO ACTING

In this chapter I have suggested that we should aspire to a binocular comprehension of persons, even though we know that, in practice, we can't achieve such binocularity any more than we can see Wittgenstein's famous figure as a duck and a rabbit at once. We should, that is, aspire to think with two lenses, no matter how much our language and psychology tempt us to think with only one. This is true whether we're thinking about the nature of persons, or the nature of technology, or the nature of nature, or, as in the next chapter, the nature of disability.

In the next chapter, I will suggest how a more binocular habit of thinking about persons can help us think in a deeper way about one form of action: the form that is embodied in the process of informed consent. Specifically, I will suggest that understanding persons first as objects and then as subjects can remind us of at least two ways in which we should show respect to persons engaged in that process. Finally, I make the move to thinking about one sort of acting: the sort where children or parents choose whether to avail themselves of an appearance-normalizing surgery.

Chapter 7

Respecting Persons as Subjects and as Objects

I suggested in chapter 5 that no one is, in principle, against "true enhancement," where a true enhancement is understood to be an intervention that promotes rather than thwarts someone's flourishing. I also suggested that the dynamics we observe in the so-called enhancement debates are much the same as the dynamics we observe in debates about virtually any form of technologically shaping selves—whether the intervention aims to improve someone's experience of her self by making her "better than normal," or "more normal," or "worse than normal," or even if the aim is to help her mock the idea of normal.

In this chapter I want to consider the class of technological interventions that helped move me beyond asking, Is it an enhancement? to asking the slightly less distracting, and what today I take to be a more salient question: Will the intervention promote or thwart someone's flourishing? Asking the latter question doesn't erase disagreements between critics of and enthusiasts about enhancement, of course. People will continue to emphasize different insights when they specify what they mean by flourishing. But, I am suggesting, at least no one should be distracted by the idea that there's something wrong, in principle, with the sorts of technological interventions I discuss in this book.

I first began to think about the particular class of technological interventions I just alluded to when I had the privilege of leading a National Endowment for the Humanities–funded working group project called Surgically Shaping Children. Over the course of three years, the working group explored surgeries that aimed at making children with atypical anatomies look "more normal." The group included surgeons, individuals who had accepted and refused appearance-normalizing surgeries, disability rights activists, and scholars from many fields including philosophy and sociology, and it considered three examples in particular: surgeries to normalize the appearance of the genitalia of children with disorders of sexual development; surgeries to normalize the appearance of children with cleft lips; and surgeries to normalize the appearance of children with unusually short limbs (that is, children with dwarfism).

In this chapter I suggest that, if we consider some important differences among those three examples, we will see why we should resist the temptation to lie down and take a rest with the principle that I am ever tempted to rest with: the principle that, instead of fixing the bodies of persons with atypical anatomies, "we" should change "their"—and "our"—minds about "their" bodies. As I trust will become clear, it is not that principle but our tendency to lie down and take a rest with it that I want to resist. I want to suggest that if we really aspire to promote the flourishing of all persons, we need a more binocular approach.

Ultimately, I will describe an informed-consent process, which draws on a binocular understanding of persons. In the first stage of the process, we treat the child and/or family as objects—in the sense that we challenge them to notice the forces that bear down on them and shape their choices. In the second stage we treat them as subjects—in the sense that, unless it is obvious that they do not have the capacity to choose, we take children and families at their word, whether they request or refuse intervention.

Before I say more about that two-stage process, however, I want to say more about the sort of "oscillating binocularity" that needs to take place in the first stage of that process. In particular, I want to say more about getting better at moving back and forth between the social and medical models of—or lenses through which to consider—disability.

MEDICAL AND SOCIAL LENSES

In the 1980s and '90s, disability theorists drew a fundamental distinction between what they called the "medical" and "social" models of disability.[1] In that first wave of disability theorizing, scholars argued that we should adopt the social model of disability, in which impairment doesn't inhere in particular traits but is created by a society that fails to accommodate people with those traits. According to the first-wave theorists, disabling traits are normatively neutral (unless they anchor a social identity, when they can be viewed as positive). As the medical sociologist Nora Groce famously observed, in the 19th century, on the small island of Martha's Vineyard, where deafness was common and everybody spoke sign language, nobody was disabled by an inability to hear.[2] The shorthand for this insight is that disabilities are "socially constructed." On the social model, impairment is a function of the social world in which the person with the trait lives. Through the social lens, the way to fix the problems that can afflict people with perceived disabilities is not to change their bodies, but to change the minds of people with typical bodies—and to change the features of the social world that are inhospitable to those who have atypical bodies.

It is hard to exaggerate the profundity of the first-wave theorists' insight. In a society that isn't scared or misapprehending of individuals who get around in wheelchairs and that provides ramps, people who get around in wheelchairs can live lives as full as anybody who gets around the typical way—just as, in a society that isn't scared or misapprehending of individuals with two X chromosomes and provides equal opportunities to all, people with two X chromosomes can flourish as well as anybody who has only one.

That profound insight, which grew out of the social model, however, was framed in terms of a stark opposition between it and the "medical" model of disability. According to the first-wave disability theorists, the medical model was the enemy of the flourishing of people with disabilities, insofar as it posited that disability was inherent in the trait. Disability wasn't constructed by an oppressive society; it was there to see, as clear as day, in the patient's body. In the medical model, the way to help people with disabilities is to change their bodies to allow them to accommodate to the dominant ways of doing things. So, whereas the social model would have people with typical bodies change their minds about the bodies of people with disabilities, the medical model would have people with typical bodies change the bodies of people with disabilities.

Fortunately, once the first-wave theorists' fundamental insight finally gained traction among scholars and even policy makers, a second wave could emerge. On the leading edge of that second wave, in the middle of the first decade of this century, Tom Shakespeare published *Disability Rights and Wrongs*,[3] in which he argued that it was time for disability rights activists (and their fellow travelers, like me) to get over what I would call the first-wave theorists' monocularity. Shortly thereafter, Jackie Leach Scully published *Disability Bioethics,*[4] which, in a very different way, made the same fundamental point. Shakespeare and Scully essentially argued that, to promote the flourishing of people with disabilities, we need—to use my jargon—at least two lenses: we need to think of disabling traits with both the social and medical models. We need to consider how "socially" constructing disabling traits differently—and how "medically" constructing (and managing) those traits—can both help promote the flourishing of people with disabilities. Before saying more about how those two lenses might together help, however, I should say just a bit about the term *normal,* which is so notoriously confounding and so unavoidable in the discussion of appearance-normalizing surgeries.

NORMALITY, AMBIGUITY, AND AMBIVALENCE

Though we use the term *normal* in many senses,[5] I want to highlight two that are especially pertinent to this discussion. We often use normal in a descriptive sense, as when we say that Abe, who is 5'11", is of normal height. We mean that Abe is somewhere in the middle of the normal height distribution for men. We can also use normal in an evaluative (or ethical or prescriptive) sense, as when we say that Bob, who is 3'11", is normal, full stop. Here we mean that Bob is inherently as good as anybody else and that, apart from his interactions with a social world created by unaccommodating others, Bob's life can go just as well—or as normally—as anybody else's.

In theory, it's harmless to notice that Bob is abnormal in the descriptive sense but normal in the evaluative one. In the world of social practice, however, we often conflate the descriptive and evaluative senses, to horrible effect—as when we conflate having a normal anatomy in the descriptive sense and being normal in the evaluative or ethical sense. We fail to remember, for example, that people whose anatomies are *ab*normal in the physical sense can be altogether normal in the ethical sense (and, of course, vice versa). Because conflating the descriptive and evaluative senses can produce such horrible effects, many thoughtful people are deeply wary of the mere mention of the ambition to attain a more normal appearance. That ambition can seem like a capitulation to the stupid, evil impulses at work in the conflation of the descriptive and evaluative senses.

Not only is the term *normal* (or *normality*) fraught with ambiguity, but our attitude toward it is deeply ambivalent. As Eva Kittay has ruefully observed, insofar as we live in a social world where to be normal in the descriptive sense is to be desirable, and insofar as we all desire to be desirable, we all desire to be normal.[6] And, as Kittay has also observed, just as strongly as we desire to be normal, we desire to be affirmed in our differences, in the ways that we are, descriptively, *ab*normal. Part of us wants to be loved, not in spite of, but because of our abnormalities. (The disability rights literature is rife with the tension between the claim that disabling traits are *distractions*, which get in the way of others seeing the person with the disabling trait, and the assumption that disabling traits are *essential constituents* of a person, which have to be embraced by the person with a disability and her peers.)

Given how ambivalent adults can be about their own normality, it is hardly surprising that they can be ambivalent about their children's. Specifically, it is hardly surprising that parents can feel torn when trying to decide whether to support or encourage normalizing interventions. On the one hand, they fervently desire normality for their children, because they believe a more normal appearance will make them accepted by and desirable to others, and thereby, they hope, help their lives go better. On the other, the idea of normalizing a child's appearance can be deeply troubling to parents, who want their child to be affirmed as she is, in her difference—in her abnormality (in the descriptive sense). As one loving parent in my Surgically Shaping Children project, the filmmaker Lisa Abelow Hedley, put it, she and her husband were acutely aware of, and determined to protect their daughter from, the "marauding conceptions of normality" at their door.[7]

THE CREATIVITY STANCE VS. THE GRATITUDE STANCE, REDUX

The particular ambivalence that parents of children with abnormal bodies face reflects a deep tension that all good parents wrestle with. And that ambivalence takes us back to the Ur tension I have discussed from the beginning of this book: between the impulse to shape and the impulse to let be, or between what I've been calling the creativity stance and the gratitude stance.

It is our responsibility as parents to shape our children. That's what traditions, schools, chores, house rules, piano lessons, sports lessons, and the like are all for. We have a conception of who we think our child should become, and we take steps that we hope will help to create that person. We think badly of parents who make no such efforts. And it is our responsibility to let our children be, to let them unfold in their own way, to let them become who they are. That's why we think badly, for example, of the violin-loving father who fails to support his football-loving son to pursue his dream or why we think badly of the ice-hockey-loving mother who fails to support her ballet-loving daughter. Children are thrown into the world with different deficits and gifts, and good parents learn how to affirm those differences, to let them be.[8]

Of course, as I discussed at length in chapter 4, means do matter ethically. Surgery and education embody different values and express different insights regarding the nature of human beings. But if we take our obligation to shape our selves and our children seriously, and if we grant that a more normal appearance can sometimes be (though, of course, is not always) a reasonable purpose to pursue, it makes it harder to give our selves the rest from thinking that goes with assuming that surgical appearance normalization is bad in itself or in principle.

Next I want to describe the three cases I mentioned above (attempting to normalize the appearance of atypical genitalia, lips, and limbs), which persuaded me that, while the purpose of normalization certainly raises ethical concerns, it is an unhelpful simplification to assume that appearance normalization is bad in principle. Frankly, that is the monocular view I clung to when I began my Surgically Shaping Children project. In retrospect, it was easy to get comfortable with that simplification because at that time I had been so focused on the very particular facts concerning the case of normalizing atypical genitalia.

CONTRASTING CASES: ATYPICAL GENITALIA AND CLEFT-LIP SURGERIES

In 1998 Alice Dreger published her germinal scholarship on the history of the treatment of people who, in the 19th century, were called "hermaphrodites."[9] Inspired at least in part by Dreger's work, people born with atypical genitalia, who then called themselves "intersexed," began to speak out. They were full of righteous

rage because, when they were infants, their parents allowed surgeons to try to normalize the appearance of their atypical
genitalia.[10]

The people speaking up charged that, to begin with, the surgeries did not succeed in achieving their purported aim of creating
genitalia that looked normal. Much worse, these surgeries often
harmed these individuals' capacity to experience sexual pleasure.
Moreover, part of the protocol was for medical professionals and
the parents to lie to and about the children: to act as if the surgical
interventions never happened. The intersex activists who spoke
out had grown up amid the shame and secrecy that surrounded
those lies.

All of which is to say that both the physiological and psychosocial consequences of these surgeries were horrific. And
I found it incredibly easy to slip from thinking that the consequences of these normalization surgeries were bad to thinking
that the normalization purpose was bad in itself. The next
case that we considered in our project, however, made me wary
of that slippage.

This was the case of surgeries aimed at normalizing the appearance of children with cleft lips. Such clefts can take very different
forms. Sometimes they entail compromised physiological functioning, such as difficulty eating or breathing, and in those cases
no one denies the appropriateness of surgical intervention.
Sometimes, however, and these were the ones my Surgically
Shaping Children project considered, the purpose of the surgery is
not to fix a physiological problem, but to make the child look more
normal. The purpose is to remove what is thought to be an obstacle
to the child's interaction with her peers. That is, the child's appearance is surgically normalized in the hopes of improving her *psychosocial* functioning.

Different from the atypical genitalia surgeries I mentioned earlier, the cleft-lip surgeries deliver what they promise: a more normal appearance. Also different from the atypical genitalia surgeries, the cleft-lip surgeries do not compromise any physiological function. Moreover, because no one tries to keep the cleft surgeries a secret, children who get them are never made to feel the shame that children with the genitalia surgeries have been made to feel.

That is, the profile of the consequences of the cleft-lip surgeries is vastly different from the profile of the consequences of the atypical genitalia surgeries. And the profile of those consequences is and should be directly pertinent to our ethical assessment.[i] When the intervention is thought to achieve its psychosocial purpose, when it actually does seem to remove an obstacle to social interaction and thus to an individual's flourishing, it becomes much harder to dismiss the intervention on the grounds that normalization is bad in itself.

To say that blanket condemnation of the normalization purpose is harder in the cleft-lip context isn't to say that even that context is always easy. In my Surgically Shaping Children project, Cassandra Aspinall, the parent of a child who was born with a cleft lip, reflected back on her reservations about letting surgeons normalize the appearance of her son's cleft lip, whose appearance,

---

i In my reflections, I am more committed to assessing consequences than are some people who are committed to invoking inviolable rights and principles, and I am more interested in inviolable rights and principles than are some people who are committed to assessing consequences. That is, I want to affirm the value of oscillating between the insights emphasized by consequentialism and deontology. *And* I want to benefit from the sorts of insights regarding human virtues and purposes, which one finds in the ethical tradition that is usually traced back to Aristotle and that today often goes under the banner of virtue ethics. I want to get better at remembering that oscillating among at least those three lenses can give deeper insight than using any one of them alone, and I want to remember that—in practice—I can't use all three in exactly the same moment.

before the surgery, she had come to love just as it was. Aspinall recalled how bad she herself felt when, as a child, she realized that her own partially repaired cleft lip triggered discomfort and distress in her beloved grandmother. Aspinall recalled asking herself when she was a child, If I'm fine with my lip in its partially repaired state, why isn't my grandmother fine with it, too?[11] For all of those misgivings, however, Aspinall now runs a clinic to support children and families making truly informed decisions about craniofacial surgeries. Like everyone else we heard from who had, or decided for her child to have, such a cleft-related intervention, Aspinall was glad she had the normalizing surgeries. Unless we can come up with a persuasive argument for why the appearance-normalization purpose is bad in this case, I think intellectual integrity requires resisting the notion that appearance normalization is bad in itself.

LIMB-LENGTHENING SURGERIES: AN EVEN MORE COMPLICATED CASE

To give a still more complex and realistic view of the clinical and human realities of appearance normalization, after considering the cases of cleft-lip and atypical genitalia surgeries, which have typically been done on infants, our Surgically Shaping Children working group considered limb-lengthening surgeries, which are done on children with dwarfism, typically when they are adolescents. These surgeries usually are done when children are 13 or 14 years old because, for physiological reasons, this is the developmental stage when maximal bone growth can be achieved.

These limb-lengthening interventions don't require mere weeks or months to recover. The process takes at least a couple of years, and it occurs in at least a couple of stages: one to lengthen the legs and the other to lengthen the arms. To initiate bone growth, a surgeon uses what is essentially a sterile hammer and chisel, and she breaks the adolescent's bone in two, thus prompting new bone tissue to grow into the gap created by the chisel. Currently, to ensure the growth of straight bones, a surgeon uses screws to attach a scaffolding device to both sides of the broken bones. Several times a day the child or her parent turns screws in the device, which pulls the broken parts of the limbs a bit farther apart, creating new space into which new bone tissue can grow. (A new technique, under investigation as I write, entails implanting a computer chip in the bones, which obviates the need for the scaffolding devices and the physical pain associated with them.)

On the spectrum of complexity among the cases we encountered, limb-lengthening surgeries and their consequences are somewhere between atypical genitalia and cleft-lip surgeries. Limb lengthening requires an enormous amount of time and a high tolerance for physical pain. The long-term physiological consequences are not as potentially horrific as those associated with some atypical genitalia surgeries, but they are not as innocuous as those associated with cleft-lip surgeries: they can entail, for example, permanent limb weakness, which limits the amount of time an individual can walk continuously.

Some people who consider their short stature to be an essential constituent of their social identity have objected to the purpose of limb-lengthening surgeries in principle. They suggest that, rather than changing their bodies, people with dwarfism and everybody else should think differently about being unusually short. Many people in our working group, including the late Paul Steven Miller, an antidiscrimination lawyer and dwarf, thought that normalization as a purpose was misguided in this context. We also had in our working group, however, a young woman, Emily Sullivan Sanford, who was born with dwarfism and who had chosen to have the limb-lengthening surgery. Sanford was perfectly frank about some of the long-term adverse physical consequences of the surgeries. Moreover, she acknowledged that she knew her mother wanted the surgery for her, and she was keenly aware of others' suspicion that she was succumbing to hateful, dominant conceptions of normality. Nonetheless, she reported in eloquent detail that she was glad that she got the surgery.[12]

Below I will discuss the thought that may now be occurring to you: "Well, yes, Sanford *said* she wanted the surgery, but that isn't what she *really* wanted; that putative desire grew out of 'false consciousness.' Of course she says she's glad she had it, but that's a rationalization."

We learned those words that come so easily to our lips—like *rationalization* and *false consciousness*—from the practitioners of the hermeneutics of suspicion, like Marx, Nietzsche, and Freud, whom I invoked in the preceding chapter. They taught us to view what people say with suspicion, to hesitate to take people at their word on the grounds that what people say they want is really a function of "no more than" the forces that bear down on them or work through them.

As important as it is to recognize the value of that interpretative strategy, so is it important to notice its limits. The hermeneutics of suspicion is as good at inviting us to question the claims of someone who says she wants a surgery as it is at inviting us to question the claims of someone who says she doesn't. It can be used to cast doubt on any claim. When I mentioned above that Paul Miller objected to the idea of the limb-lengthening surgeries (which were not available when he was a child) you could suggest that he was "in denial" about what being a dwarf was really like for him. You could suggest that he was just rationalizing his experience.

To observe that the hermeneutics of suspicion can be used to raise questions about the manifest content of virtually any claim is not to deny the seriousness of those questions. It does help explain, though, why I will suggest below that there is a time for a hermeneutics of suspicion and a time for taking people at their word.

In describing the different facts concerning the different surgeries, I have sought to suggest that, when we consider the consequences of these surgeries (for example, different levels of success at achieving their stated aim, different levels of adverse effects, etc.) the normalization purpose can increase or decrease in salience. As the physiological and psychosocial costs of some atypical genitalia surgeries came to be gigantic, the persuasiveness of the normalization critique also grew. With cleft-lip surgeries, where the physiological and psychosocial costs are negligible, the critique of normalization has less traction.

Even if I do so warily and reluctantly, I cannot but endorse the normalization purpose in the cleft-lip case; given the way we appear to be wired and socialized, reducing such an anatomical difference is an instance of us using our creativity to promote someone's flourishing. And the physiological and psychosocial consequences of limb-lengthening are so mixed that I am willing to accept that reasonable people will reach different conclusions. Which ultimately is to say—at the risk of being hopelessly boring—that, if we want to promote the flourishing of real people, we need to promote a process of truly informed consent, where the human beings who will live with the choice receive help weighing all of the consequences associated with the normalization purpose.

WHO GETS TO CHOOSE—AND WHEN?

In the cases I discuss here, that question is even more complicated than usual. Even more than adults, children have to be understood as individuals and as members of families.[13] As members of families, children are, for much of their early lives, the beneficiaries (or victims) of choices made for them by their parents or guardians. Of course, another thing that makes the who-gets-to-choose question so complex in this context is that children's capacity to participate in decision making about their own care changes over time.

At least since 1995, the American Academy of Pediatrics (AAP) has suggested that patients "should participate in decision making commensurate with their development."[14] As a general matter, according to the AAP, in the case of infants and very young children, parents have to give "informed permission" for an intervention; they decide for infants. In the case of older school-age children, clinicians are expected to get the child's "assent" and the parents' "informed permission." Further, the AAP suggests that adolescents can in principle sometimes give informed consent. According to the AAP (and according to the working group I led), as a child's capacity to participate in the decision grows, so should the weight of what she says she does or doesn't want.

As my Surgically Shaping Children working group also suggested, as the physiological and psychosocial costs of the surgeries grow, so does the importance of waiting to involve the child in the decision. Deciding without a child about cleft-lip surgeries may be perfectly reasonable, whereas deciding about "cosmetic" atypical genitalia surgeries is not, as long as the potential costs associated with such surgeries are enormous. It is imperative to involve children in a decision about an intervention with as mixed a profile of consequences as the one associated with limb lengthening, and it is imperative to remember that reasonable people will reach different conclusions in such hard cases.

To say that we should expect reasonable disagreements is not to say that we should accept mistakes. It is as important to try to distinguish the two, as it is to remember that the line between them is not nearly as bright as we would wish. The most fundamental mistake is for anyone involved in the decision-making process to allow anything other than the child's flourishing to be paramount. In particular, it is a mistake if parents (or physicians) allow their anxiety about the child's difference to overwhelm their estimation of what surgery can and can't achieve. Based on anecdotal evidence, it is my impression that some of the surgeons who once offered to surgically normalize the appearance of the faces of children with Down syndrome have stopped, because they discovered that their interventions were not improving the psychosocial functioning of these children. They appear to have discovered that, essentially, they had been operating on the children's bodies to reduce the parents' anxiety.[ii] Surely, any surgery that compromised sexual functioning—as surgeries on atypical genitalia have—would also qualify as a mistake.

Just as requests for surgery can be based on mistakes, the same goes for refusals. It would, for example, be a mistake for a parent to let her opposition to normalization in principle allow her to ignore how a particular normalization could promote her child's flourishing. Refusing cleft-lip surgery for one's child on the grounds that it would send her the harmful message that she isn't okay the way she is,[15] might grow out of the noblest of principles, but would, I believe,

---

ii This is what I was told by a representative of an association of American cosmetic surgeons when I tried—without success—to find a surgeon who would be willing to speak to my Surgically Shaping Children group about such surgeries.

nonetheless be a mistake. We should not sacrifice the flourishing of children on the altar of any principle, not even the noble principle of affirming anatomical difference.

REASONABLE REQUESTS AND REFUSALS

Recognizing that reasonable people can reach different conclusions, of course, requires us to learn to respect both refusals of and requests for intervention. Consider the case of a 15-year-old girl I'll call Molly, who was born not with a cleft lip but with other highly atypical craniofacial differences. Molly was marvelously articulate in her request for surgeries that would normalize the appearance of her face:

> I don't want to have this [craniofacial] surgery for a medical reason; I want to do this because I don't want to look so different that people stare or think that I have a developmental problem. . . . I still want to look like me and I was afraid the surgery would change who I was because I really like myself. My mom told me it didn't matter if I decided to have the surgery or not. She said what I looked like on the outside could never change the person I am on the inside. That made me feel better. . . . [But having the surgery] will make it easier for people to get to know me instead of just looking at my outside.[16]

Apparently, it doesn't take a PhD to understand arguments from the goals of medicine or to deploy the concept of authenticity. Molly understands that the purpose of the surgery is to fix a psychosocial, not a physiological, problem. She likes herself as she is, and she even worries that, insofar as how she looks is part of who she is, the surgery would change who she is and thus is troubling. (Unlike many of her elders, she can use two lenses almost at once: she takes her atypical features to be a distraction and an important element of who she is.) All things considered, she says she wants the surgery, to make it easier for others to get to know who she thinks she really is.

Here again critics of technologically shaping our selves have a chance to apply a hermeneutics of suspicion: "Well, Molly *says* she wants intervention, but she doesn't really. She has internalized the ideal of normality that she would reject if she could see clearly." Once again, however, I ask you to notice how equally easy it is to invoke such a hermeneutics of suspicion to cast doubt on a *refusal* of surgery.

Harilyn Russo, a psychotherapist and influential disability rights activist, was born with cerebral palsy, which makes her way of moving through the world atypical. She has described the feeling of being assaulted by her own mother's attempts to normalize her ways of moving when she was a child. That is, she has described the experience of having her desire to refuse intervention egregiously ignored.

[My mother] made numerous attempts over the years of my childhood to have me go for physical therapy and to practice walking more "normally" at home. I vehemently refused all her efforts....My disability, with my different walk and talk and my involuntary movements, having been with me all of my life, was part of me, part of my identity. With these disability features, I felt complete and whole. My mother's attempt to change my walk, strange as it may seem, felt like an assault on myself, an incomplete acceptance of all of me, an attempt to make me over.[17]

Different from Molly, Ms. Russo felt no ambivalence about appearance normalization, and she had no patience for the idea that appearance normalization would let others get to know her. For her, appearance normalization felt like a rejection of who she really was. She viewed normalization as an attempt to separate her from her self, from who she really is. It seemed an assault on her wholeness, a form of enforced alienation.

Of course, the observer who thinks it is obvious that Ms. Russo would benefit from a more normal appearance can say, "Well, she *says* she didn't and doesn't want normalization, but that's because she's 'in denial.' She says her anatomical abnormality makes her whole, or who she really is, but she's lying to herself. It's a coping mechanism."

Like the patient's language of authenticity, the observer's hermeneutics of suspicion can be used to support *or* criticize intervention. This makes for a far more complex situation than any of us would wish. Our ethical deliberations would be much simpler if we could either just take people at their word when they say an intervention will or won't allow them to become whole—or we could refuse to take people at their word on the grounds that we understand the forces acting on them better than they do, and thus understand better than they do what's good for them. A harder, better strategy, though, seeks to integrate the best of what's at work in applying a hermeneutics of suspicion (and, as it were, seeing through people's words) and in taking people at their word. In such a strategy, I will suggest, we benefit from the binocular understanding of persons I mentioned earlier, seeing them first as objects and then as subjects. The notion of considering persons first through one lens and then through another is not as foreign as it might sound at first. In fact, anyone familiar with the two major stages of a criminal law proceeding is already familiar with a strategy that is in an important respect similar.

A WAY IN WHICH COURTS ADOPT
A BINOCULAR VIEW OF PERSONS

In the context of criminal law, we are accustomed to thinking of the defendant first as a subject and then as an object, in the following sense. If someone is accused of a capital crime, it is assumed that she can stand trial, unless it can be demonstrated that she was coerced by someone or something. The judge and jury understand the sense in which the defendant was acted on by myriad bio-psycho-social forces when she did (or didn't do) what she's accused of. But in the first phase of the trial, in which it is determined whether the defendant is guilty, the judge and jury bracket their knowledge of the sense in which the defendant is an object. The jury is required to see the defendant through the subject lens—as someone who was free to choose—and to determine whether she did what she has been accused of.

In the second, penalty phase of a trial for a capital crime, the jury is invited to see the defendant as an object—in the sense that they are invited to consider the forces that bore down on the defendant, whether her abusive childhood or her brain tumor. A consideration of such forces can mitigate or aggravate her penalty.

That is, because it is as hard to think of persons as subjects and as objects at the same time as it is to see Wittgenstein's figure as a rabbit and a duck at once, the criminal law offers a two-step strategy. I am of course speaking quite schematically here,[iii] but there is a sense in which such proceedings give the judge and jury an opportunity to think of the defendant first as a subject who was

---

iii For an account of how genetic or neuroscientific evidence might one day influence thinking about that first, guilt phase of a trial, see Paul Appelbaum, "The Double Helix Takes the Witness Stand: Behavioral and Neuropsychiatric Genetics in Court," *Neuron* 82 (2014), http://dx.doi.org/10.1016/j.neuron.2014.05.026.33333.

free to choose how she acted, and then as an object whose actions were determined by myriad bio-psycho-social forces. As we are about to see, in the clinical context, too, there is a way in which it can help to view persons as objects and as subjects. In this context, though, it helps to reverse the order, seeing people first as objects and then second as subjects.

CHALLENGING PROVIDERS AND FAMILIES AT THE BEGINNING OF THE DAY

I am suggesting that it can be useful to think of a process of truly informed consent as entailing at least two stages. At the beginning of the day, it is important for patients to be helped to think of themselves as objects: as beings whose views are determined by the myriad forces that bear down on them. Please notice that, insofar as both the medical and social models of disability offer different *explanations* of the source and nature of the difficulties that people with disabilities experience, both of those lenses can help us consider persons as objects. The two lenses give different insights into the forces acting on people with disabilities—and remind us of the different forces that can be recruited to promote the understanding and flourishing of those same people.

It isn't just patients who are affected by myriad forces beneath or beyond their consciousness, and who would benefit from using a hermeneutics of suspicion to consider the forces that shape their views. At the beginning of the day, health care providers, too, have to be willing to apply a hermeneutics of suspicion to their own views. To see why, it helps to consider what was once called the "disability paradox."[18] What was taken to be "paradoxical" is the fact that people with disabilities consistently report that the quality of their lives is better than what healthy providers would have predicted.[19] That is, healthy providers (and others) consistently "underestimate the self-reported well-being of people with disabilities and serious illness."[20] They fail to understand the extent to which we can all adapt to atypical circumstances far better than we imagine.[21] That is why the physicians and disability scholars Sunil Kothari and Kirsti Kirschner suggest a respect in which we should "abandon the golden rule"[22]: we can get into all manner of trouble when we assume we can put ourselves in the shoes of the other. Kothari and Kirschner are saying that, though people who don't live with a disability think they know what they would want if they did live with a disability, they don't.

A HERMENEUTICS OF SUSPICION CAN USE THE SOCIAL AND MEDICAL LENSES

If, for example, parents come to a physician, saying they want limb lengthening for their child with dwarfism, in the belief that the surgery will promote her flourishing, it is important to challenge that idea. Essentially, parents and children should be helped to explore the questions they are probably already asking: Do we really want this? What are the destructive social norms that are pushing us to choose this painful and potentially dangerous set of operations? Have we fully understood the ways in which people with dwarfism have flourished with their bodies just as they were thrown into the world with them? Have we considered the option to refuse surgery seriously enough?

If, for example, a child or family says they do not want an intervention, on the grounds that accepting it would be to capitulate to "marauding conceptions of normal," then this belief, too, should be challenged. If, for example, a family says, "We have come to love our child just as she is, with her abnormal anatomy just as it is," the medical professionals and anyone else who is part of the conversation should be prepared to challenge that view, asking, "Have you considered all of the respects in which intervening surgically might promote your child's flourishing?"

The aim of these beginning-of-the-day conversations is not for medical professionals or anyone else to persuade families or patients of a particular choice. It is to facilitate the family's or patient's thinking about the meaning of the alternatives. Professionals do this by inviting families and patients to oscillate between lenses they find more and less congenial. When, for example, it comes to understanding disabling traits, some families or patients will find the social lens more congenial, and others the medical; the point is to help patients benefit from the insights of both.

DETERMINING WHETHER A DECISION IS TRULY INFORMED

At the end of this first stage in the process of truly informed consent, professionals need to ask if the person who is supposed to benefit from the process has benefited from it. They need to determine if the patient or family is ready to move to the second stage. I don't imagine there is a foolproof way to assess whether a family has succeeded in thinking through the meaning of the alternatives, but some basic questions can help assess whether it has failed.

Professionals must ask, Is the child mature enough to be involved in the decision, and, if so, has she been heard?[23] As

Priscilla Alderson and others have documented, children can understand their predicaments much better than some professionals and parents imagine.[24] Professionals must also ask, Can the parents see beyond their own anxieties about the child's future to what will actually promote the child's flourishing? Both of those questions are essentially trying to get to the most basic question of all: Do these children and parents understand the relevant facts and their own value commitments well enough to make a truly informed decision?

If the relevant team of medical professionals determines that the answer to that question is no, then it is time to get additional help. This is a situation where someone trained in clinical bioethics, or even a bioethics committee, may provide assistance. But if the answer is yes, if the family is capable of making as truly informed a decision as any of us can ever make, then it is time to move to the second stage.

TAKING PEOPLE AT THEIR WORD, AT THE END OF THE DAY

If at the beginning of the day we show someone respect by challenging her intuitions about the best path, at the end of the day we show respect by deferring to her truly informed choice. At the end of the day, that is, we have to take people at their word. We make the transition from thinking of them as objects that are acted on by all sorts of forces beyond their immediate consciousness, to thinking of them as subjects who are as free as any of us ever is in making a choice.

Taking people at their word will sometimes mean deferring to decisions that surprise us. It requires being prepared to defer to

refusals of and requests for technological intervention. At the end
of the day, some patients will, invoking the insights of the social
lens, choose to refuse intervention—as Ms. Russo presumably
would have done, had she been listened to as a child. Some patients
will, invoking the insights offered by the medical lens, choose to
request intervention—as Molly did.

IMPORTANT CAVEAT

You may have just noticed the way in which *the social lens* can be
especially useful for someone who proceeds from *the gratitude
stance* and who wants to give an account of her *refusal* of surgical
intervention. And you may have noticed the way in which *the medical lens* can be especially useful for someone who proceeds from
the creativity stance and who wants to give an account of her *request*
for surgical intervention. While these patterns of alignment among
stance, lens, and decision are common in the class of technologically shaping selves debates I've discussed in this book, it is essential to notice that these patterns are not the same even just across
all of the debates concerning technologies and children.

Consider a set of debates that I have not broached in this
book: the ones concerning whether to use advanced technologies
to save the life of a profoundly imperiled newborn. Here, a family
who wants to request aggressive technological intervention to
keep their newborn alive can employ *the social lens*, through which
what is hardest about disabling traits inheres not in the traits but in
how they are constructed by unaccommodating societies. They
can, adopting *the creativity stance*, remind us that it is our job as
human beings to creatively transform our selves and the world. In
this context, a family who wants to refuse aggressive technological

intervention and to allow their profoundly imperiled newborn to die can employ the medical lens—in the sense of what disability scholars call "the medical model of disability." That is, the family who wants to refuse treatment can invoke the respect in which what's hard about disability traits isn't socially constructed but inheres in those traits. They can, adopting *the gratitude stance*, remind us that it is our job as human beings to let things be, in this case, to let nature take its course.

That is, the social lens might be deployed in the debates about normalizing children's appearances to *refuse* technological intervention and might be used in the debates about imperiled newborns to *request* intervention. The medial lens, too, could be used to refuse or request intervention. Though, as I discussed in earlier chapters, we can't help but notice patterns of alignments among stances, lenses, and decisions, and though it would make our intellectual lives easier if those patterns were more stable, they are not—not even, as I will discuss more in the last part of the book, within the same debates.

A MONOCULAR MOMENT IN
A BINOCULAR PROCESS

There is an important sense in which, at the end of the day, the sort of oscillating between lenses that occurs in deeper thinking has to stop. If decent action is what we're after, we have to take a break from thinking. Indeed, there is a sense in which, at the end of the day, the patient's decision will be *monocular*. Our action can reflect the benefit of oscillating between stances and lenses, but in the end we can make one decision only. Because we can't refuse and request the same intervention, there is a sense in which making a decision will constitute a monocular moment.

If, though, that moment comes at the end of a process that is binocular in the ways I've described, we will be amply prepared to be surprised by choices that others make—both choices to request and to refuse technological interventions. Such an understanding can help prepare us to accept that people proceeding from different stances, using different lenses, will in some hard cases reach different but equally respect-worthy decisions. To use language that the philosopher Isaiah Berlin used in a different context, talk of truly informed consent is not "the stuff of which calls to heroic action" is made. But as he might also say, "If there is some truth in the view, perhaps that is sufficient."[25]

Closing Thoughts

When I entered the field of bioethics in the early 1990s, I encountered in some of the colleagues I most respected what we might call, borrowing from the neuroscientist Antonio Damasio, a "high reason"[1] view of bioethics. On such a view, which had infused wide swaths of the field since its inception in the late 1960s and early '70s, bioethicists impartially applied reason to answer hard ethical questions. Such a view of how reason worked wasn't held by bioethicists only. At about the same time that bioethics came into being, psychologists like Lawrence Kohlberg were advancing the notion that the ultimate achievement of human development was to impartially apply universal principles of reason to questions of justice.[2] Surely not all bioethicists shared what I call here the high-reason view, but the promise of expertly applying reason to answer hard ethical questions helped garner attention and funding for the fledgling field.

As a reader of Aeschylus, Shakespeare, and Dostoyevsky, not to mention Marx, Nietzsche, and Freud, I was skeptical about the high-reason view of human beings, and thus of bioethics. But as a newcomer to the field, I was eagerly open to new, clearer ways of thinking. So, as I described in chapter 1, when I embarked on my first major project at The Hastings Center, I sought to build an argument "against enhancement" based on reason alone.

As I also described in my opening chapter, over time I came to recognize the extent to which my ethical conclusion regarding the badness of enhancement grew out of more than reason alone. Among other things, it grew out of a deep feeling or intuition about what the appropriate stance toward our selves and the world is. Making the case against enhancement was not, or at least was not only, impartially applying reason to a hard problem. It was finding reasons to support a conclusion that felt right and that I began with.[3]

Moreover, I can now see the extent to which defending my position against enhancement was tantamount to defending my way of being in the world: a way that is, among other things, slow, reflective, and eager to find goodness even in some of the features of the world that at first seem hard—a way that is eager to learn to let things be. It's not that reason played no role in my argument against enhancement, nor that feeling played the only role. It's that the reasons that seemed most salient had everything to do with my stance, with my felt sense of my proper attitude toward, and place in, the world.

I surely am *not* saying that feelings have any sort of otherwise inaccessible moral authority. Nor am I saying that we can't ever distinguish between better and worse reasons. Nor am I saying that we should rely on, or defer to, feelings. I simply am saying that it is a failure of reason to disregard the role that feeling plays in determining the reasons that seem most salient to us—to all of us, even those of us who take ourselves to be especially committed to reason. I am saying that, as citizens of democracies, we owe each other reasons for our positions *and* we owe it to ourselves and each other to recognize that the reasons that seem most salient to us depend, in part, on the stance toward the world that we feel most comfortable in. We owe it to each other to strive for impartiality—and to recognize our ineluctable partiality.

As I also described in chapter 1, the more fully I noticed the role of feeling and intuition at work on my side of the so-called enhancement debate, the more fully I could notice and acknowledge the insights on the other. The other side was emphasizing insights I had ignored or denied, not because they had nothing going for them, but because I wanted to win a point. Over time, I came to appreciate the way in which understanding the question could be more intellectually satisfying, if less exciting, than trying to win the point. I could go from speaking as if I was against enhancement to asking about enhancement—about what true enhancement is. I could go from answering the question, Are you for or against enhancement? to asking the question concerning the meaning of enhancement: What is "true" enhancement? What is the difference between an intervention that would thwart someone's flourishing and one that would promote it?

The upside of that approach is that I got to reduce the bad sort of anxiety associated with telling half the story, and I also got to deepen my understanding of the question at hand. The downside is that, because there are no crisp or final or expert answers to such meaning questions, I had to give up the fantasy of being able to dispense the sorts of answers that some people hoped and thought I, as a bioethicist, could offer.

To say that there are no crisp answers to the question concerning the meaning of enhancement is not to say that we can or should throw up our hands in the face of the practical ethical questions. Just as much as our commitment to truth requires recognizing the partiality of our answers to meaning questions, our commitment to justice requires giving answers to practical ethical questions. Just as much as we should be wary of intellectual laziness masquerading as moral courage, we should be wary of moral cowardice masquerading as intellectual rigor.

I have suggested that, to grapple with that fundamental tension between our commitments to truth and to justice—between the demands in the two epigraphs I placed at the beginning of this book—a binocular approach can be helpful. More specifically, I have suggested that the notion of oscillating binocularity can help us envision a process of thinking about meaning questions that don't admit of final answers, and I have suggested that a binocular understanding of persons can help us conceive of the process whereby we make practical decisions in a clinical context. In the remainder of these closing thoughts, I want to say just a bit more about what I mean by those two suggestions.

MEANING QUESTIONS
AND OSCILLATING BINOCULARITY

As I suggested in chapter 3, the notion of oscillating binocularity can help us resist the temptation to make a big binary choice and speak as if we were for or against technologically shaping our selves, full stop. I suggested that in the privacy of our own thinking we already do shuttle back and forth between the insights associated with the creativity stance, which emphasizes our ethical obligation to shape our selves and the world, and the gratitude stance, which emphasizes our ethical obligation to let our selves and the world be. I suggested that, while one stance will feel more comfortable than the other, none of us who is thoughtful will feel comfortable in only one. The notion of oscillating binocularity is supposed to help us remember that we should get better at doing publicly what we already do in the privacy of our most concerted efforts to understand: shuttle between the insights harbored in the creativity and gratitude stances.

I also intend the notion of oscillating binocularity to help us resist the temptation to make the smaller binary choices that are required when we try to defend a conclusion for or against. In chapters 3, 4, and 5, I gave examples of some of the binary choices between particular lenses that enthusiasts and critics can enlist when they try to win their point. I described how, for example, from the creativity stance, human beings tend to look to be creators, whereas from the gratitude stance we tend to look to be creatures; how from the creativity stance, nature tends to look to be a mechanism that we can engineer to suit our ends, whereas from the gratitude stance it tends to look to be a fragile web that we endanger with our efforts at engineering; and how from the creativity stance technology tends to look to be a value-free tool that we can use to shape our selves in ways we freely choose, whereas from the gratitude stance technology looks to be a value-laden frame that shapes our choices and ultimately our selves.

In chapter 6 I considered a different binary choice that our language puts to us when we attempt to talk about what human beings are—either we are objects or we are subjects—and I suggested that we can and should see our selves with both lenses. We are objects, whose behaviors can be explained from the third-person perspective of natural and social science; we are constituted by the same forces and subjected to the same laws as are all of the other objects in the universe—even though we are unique among animals in the extent to which reasons can be part of the causal chain that explains our behaviors. We are also subjects, the sites of subjective experience; we are the animals who have and share feelings and reasons about being in the world. To understand this feature of our selves, we have to listen to what individual human beings say it is like to be them. What we see through the subject lens, when we try to understand what someone's first-person experience is like for her, isn't illusory or epi-phenomenal, and it surely is not inferior to what we see through the object lens, from the third-person perspective. It is different in kind.

To comprehend persons in depth, we need to oscillate between the two lenses. Settling down with the object lens alone (as some neuroscientists are wont to do) and settling down with the subject lens alone (as some humanists are wont to do) are equally symptoms of what I have called the bad sort of monocularity, the sort born not of moral integrity but of intellectual lassitude. To paraphrase the book's first epigraph, if we want the truth to stand clear before us, we have to, for as long as possible, resist the temptation to choose between lenses or stances.

RESISTING THE TEMPTATION TO MAKE A CONCEPTUAL LEDGER WITH NEATLY ARRAYED BINARIES

In chapter 7 we discovered how using the subject and object lenses comes naturally to both enthusiasts and critics. At one juncture of these debates, *critics* of surgically shaping children emphasize that we are *objects*, with myriad forces bearing down on us, which make us think we want interventions that we really don't. At the same juncture in the debate, *enthusiasts* emphasize that we are *subjects*, who are perfectly capable of freely discerning what we really do and don't want. It is essential to notice, however, that at a different juncture in the same debates, *critics* will emphasize that we are *subjects*—as when they emphasize that, because we are reason-giving creatures, we should use reasons to change our minds about someone's atypical body rather than, say, use a scalpel to change that body. At that same juncture in the debate, *enthusiasts* will emphasize that because we are *objects*, because we are mechanisms that admit of technological fixing, it is mere prejudice to prefer reasons to scalpels. (In that chapter we also noticed that enthusiasts and critics can, in different arguments, appeal to different lenses on disability.)

Here I am getting at what I take to be a fundamental point: as tempting as it may be, we have to resist the idea that we can, as it were, line up the relevant binaries along two sides of a single ledger, with perhaps "creativity" being the heading for one column and "gratitude" the heading for the other. Yes, at various points in the debates, it may be possible to array some binaries (as I did at some points in chapters 3, 4, and 5) in such a way. But such an array won't accurately depict the conceptual situation for long, and as a result, it won't get us very far. A single-ledger approach, no matter how tempting, would entail absurd simplification. Like our desire for one lens, our desire for one ledger is as understandable as it is doomed to fail in helping us achieve the understanding we need.

ONTOLOGICAL VERSUS EPISTEMOLOGICAL DISTINCTIONS

To elaborate my claim that a binocular understanding of persons helps us think about the process we should use to reach decisions in the clinical context, it can help to distinguish between two sorts of distinction. Insofar as ontology is about the nature of the beings that exist, I have been making an ontological distinction when I have suggested that human beings are objects and are subjects. Insofar as epistemology is about the nature of what we can know, the distinction between our knowledge of objective facts regarding the world and our subjective preferences regarding it is epistemological. It is one thing to distinguish between persons as subjects and as objects (the ontological distinction) and another to distinguish between the subjective preferences of persons and the objective facts concerning their situation (the epistemological distinction).[4]

The ontological-epistemological distinction may seem tedious at first, but it can help clarify what I meant when I claimed that a binocular understanding of persons can help us conceive of the process of truly informed consent. Insofar as the ontological distinction reminds us that we are subjects and are objects, it reminds us that our subjectivity (the fact that we are subjects) and our "objectivity" (here referring to the fact that we are objects) are equally important features of the world and deserve equal attention and honor. The epistemological distinction, on the other hand, reminds us that sometimes our subjective preferences should be honored and sometimes should not be. Sometimes our subjective preferences reflect an atypical experience of or attitude toward our selves or the world, and sometimes they reflect a mistake in our understanding of our selves or the world. Sometimes our subjective preferences reflect a reasonable disagreement about how to interpret the objective facts and sometimes they reflect a mistake about the facts. We can be prepared to honor the truly informed request of a person with dwarfism for limb-lengthening surgery, and we can also be prepared to refuse to honor the request of a person with anorexia, who, on the verge of dying, says she doesn't want to eat because she is fat.

A BINOCULAR UNDERSTANDING
OF PERSONS AND
ONE SORT OF PRACTICAL QUESTION

No matter how important it is to learn to oscillate between the myriad pairs of lenses we need for thinking about meaning questions, we can't refuse to choose sides forever—not, anyway, if we aspire to make practical ethical decisions about how to act, and not if we aspire to exhibit moral integrity. As the second epigraph of the book reminds us, living decently requires that we sometimes choose sides.

Fortunately, we can, as I discussed in the preceding chapter, engage in a process of practical decision making that itself reflects a binocular understanding of our selves. At least in the clinical context, I have been suggesting, we can think of the informed-consent process as requiring us first to treat each other as objects, with myriad forces bearing down on us, determining our preferences, and then second, with rare exceptions, we treat each other as subjects who can freely choose.

As I also discussed in the preceding chapter, in that first step of the process, at the beginning of the day, we show each other respect by challenging each other to oscillate between the myriad pairs of lenses on offer, and we thereby help each other to explore the meaning questions that are always in the background of such practical decisions. It is at the end of the first step, at the end of the beginning of the day, when we need to remember the ever-elusive epistemological distinction between objective facts and subjective preferences. Secular, liberal pluralists like me are deeply wary of ever suggesting that we know better than someone else what is good for her. Our epistemological humility attunes us to the enormous danger of failing to defer to an individual's choice. We are exquisitely aware of the danger associated with saying that we know that someone else is making a mistake about the nature of her own experience or about what will truly promote her flourishing.

At the same time, we are, or should be, equally aware of the danger of failing to muster the epistemological confidence to say exactly that. As Isaiah Berlin, Martha Nussbaum, Amy Gutmann, Jonathan Glover, and many others have observed,[5] if we fail to muster the epistemological confidence to attempt to distinguish between subjective reports on experience and the objective facts concerning such experience, we give up an essential tool for criticizing injustice. If we aspire to speak up for those who are deprived of their right to flourish, we must be prepared to own up to our belief that we know some "objective" facts about what human flourishing consists in.

Perhaps the most fundamental of those facts is that, if we are to flourish, we cannot be in chains, literally or figuratively. It is upon the claim to such knowledge that we reject the assertion of the slave who reports that she is content in her servitude. It is on that basis that we refuse to interpret an abjectly impoverished and overtly oppressed person's "lack of grieving and lamentation"[6] to be a true indication that she is flourishing. And, ultimately, it is on that basis that we reject the assertion of the parent of the child with atypical genitalia, who says that more normal-appearing genitalia will be more important for that child than genitalia that function normally. We know that human flourishing requires some basic opportunities and capacities to be in place, among them the capacity to experience sexual pleasure. That parent, as much as the slave or the person who is otherwise overtly oppressed, is making a mistake, and it is here that a hermeneutics of suspicion can serve justice. Of course, a hermeneutics of suspicion can also serve injustice. Just think of the immeasurable human misery caused by the claim that people who say they want to have sex with people of the same gender don't really want that. There is no foolproof way to know when one's hermeneutics of suspicion will serve justice or injustice.

In the vast majority of cases, where the person facing a decision about technologically shaping her self demonstrates that she has the capacity to choose as much as any of us ever does, then after that first step of challenging her, it will be time to move on. It will be time to stop with the hermeneutics of suspicion and with trying to see through what she says and to start taking seriously the surface of what she is saying, to take what she is saying at face value. That is, it will be time for the second step, when we treat each other as subjects and take each other at our words. We show each other respect by deferring to each other's truly informed choices, and we gird ourselves to be surprised by people making decisions that we imagine we would not make for ourselves. There are, for example, people with disabilities who want a normalizing intervention, as well as people with disabilities who don't.

As I have already allowed, there is a sense in which recommending a process of truly informed consent is deeply boring. Achieving truly informed consent, however, is anything but. It takes courage to challenge each other and confidence to, in rare circumstances, say that someone is making a mistake, as when a parent requests a surgery for her child that is really to treat the parent's own discomfort. And it takes humility to defer to someone who makes a choice we can't imagine making for ourselves—to remember that none of us has expert answers to the meaning questions that are always in the background of such a decision.

OBSERVATIONS AND CAVEATS
CONCERNING *BINOCULARITY*

First, if binocularity entails using two lenses at once, and if when I have referred to binocular thinking or binocular understanding I have referred to using one lens and then another, the term *binocularity* may seem inapt. Wouldn't something like "serial *monocularity*" be more apt? I don't think so. Yes, it is true that we just are not built for seeing with two lenses at once any more than we are wired to see Wittgenstein's figure as a rabbit and duck at once. But, as I have said from the beginning, I don't intend the metaphor of binocularity to name an achievement or to be a panacea. I intend it only to name an aspiration to a habit of thinking that can deepen our understanding and contribute to, though, of course, cannot ensure, better action.

Second, while I hope that my discussion of the informed-consent process is relevant to the practical world of the clinic, I have said very little that is directly relevant to the practical world of public policy making. I do, however, think that a more binocular approach could be useful in that context, too. It does seem to me that people called bioethicists, in virtue of their handle on the history of ethical theories, their handle on the scientific or technological facts of the matter, their understanding of the history of the relevant policy debates, their understanding of the nature of policy debates in general, and their experience with welcoming and probing multiple perspectives, can help facilitate public conversations about the ethical and social implications of emerging science and technology. Bioethicists can help others with less experience resist lapsing into the monocularity that tempts all of us all of the time, and that is perhaps nowhere more tempting than in the context of public policy debates regarding new technologies.

I'm reassured to know that I'm not alone in thinking that bioethicists need to be wary of appearing to be in possession of expert answers to at least some sorts of public policy questions.[i] The President's Council on Bioethics, for example, which had critical things to say about the prospect of "enhancement technologies," and Neil Levy, for example, who had enthusiastic things to say about the same prospect, refrain from offering policy advice when it comes to enhancement. They both, wisely I believe, resisted the temptation to make public policy pronouncements about "enhancement technologies." Both even use the same phrase to communicate their understanding of their task; both say they aspire to do no more nor less than help us go into the future "with our eyes open."[7] They both speak, that is, as lovers of truth: trying to articulate issues regarding the meaning of enhancement, not offering an ethical pronouncement. Again, if we bioethicists remember that we don't possess expert answers concerning the meaning questions that will always be in the background of the practical decisions made at the level of policy, I think we can and should play a role. But when we do, we are obligated to ward off the wizard fantasy, which others can have about us even more than we have it about ourselves.

Third, I hope that in my attempt to give the creativity stance its due, I didn't fail to give the gratitude stance its due as well. It does seem to me that, at least in the United States today, gratitude is more in need of support than creativity. Learning to let some

---

i As I have observed before, it is perfectly reasonable to distinguish between questions about which there *are* expert answers (e.g., is climate change real?) and questions about which there are *not* (e.g., what is true enhancement?).

things be may be one of the hardest problems to which we need to apply our ability to think creatively. Letting things be may always have been, and likely will be from here on out, a hard sell. For starters, there just isn't the kind of money to be made in letting things be as there is in transforming things. If we in the United States suffer from a status quo bias, it may be a bias toward the notion that the more we creatively transform ourselves and the world the better. For all that is marvelous in our ability to do just that, we have to get better at grappling with the ways in which such transformations cannot alone make us happier.[8] That insight is as familiar and obvious as it is hard to act in accordance with. My lack of attention to the role of money in the debates about using technology to shape our selves is an important lacuna, which I hope others will energetically fill.

My final observation has to do with my reliance on a binary distinction that has undergirded my entire exploration and that I have yet to criticize. From the beginning, I have pitted *understanding* some question against *winning* the debate regarding that question. I have, that is, spoken at times as if the desire to understand and the desire to win are in binary opposition. To be fair, I have from the beginning acknowledged that some questions have to be answered—and that justice can demand that we fight to see our side win. But there is a way in which I may have lapsed into a sort of "monocularity" of the bad sort, in the sense of intellectual laziness. Specifically, in thumping for the value of one "lens" (understanding), I may have failed to duly appreciate the other (winning).

To appreciate that the desire to win can conduce to, rather than undermine, understanding, one doesn't have to hearken back to the Nietzschean idea that understanding emerges only out of a contest. The philosophers Dan Sperber and Hugo Mercier have observed that, while it is true that individuals use reason primarily to win arguments, the end result is deeper understanding for the group.[9] That is, while individuals may use reason more to win than to understand, the aggregate effect over time is increased understanding within the group. Sperber and Mercier would predict, I think, that individual critics and enthusiasts fighting to win their points regarding technologically shaping our selves will ultimately conduce to the group's deeper understanding.

I think that something like that has actually happened in the context of the so-called enhancement debates. It may even be fair to say that we have entered what we might call a second wave of those debates, where we're getting better at talking about what true enhancement is, rather than arguing for or against it. I, of course, take my own work to be an example of this kind of progress. From the enthusiastic side there seem to be several notable examples, including Allen Buchanan's recommendation of a "balanced approach" to enhancement;[10] John Harris's articulation of a worry that some interventions being hailed as moral enhancements aren't really "worthy of the name";[11] and James Hughes's acknowledgment of "the internal contradictions" of the Enlightenment that haunt the enthusiastic movement called transhumanism.[12]

At a minimum, over time we have been able to achieve considerable consensus on some forms of self-shaping that are beyond the pale and some forms that a decent society should provide. As I have suggested, nobody is for Brave New World's Soma, and nobody is against using new technologies that enable someone to act in the world as she really is and as the world really is. As we keep the conversation going about what true human enhancement means, it will no doubt be important to give understanding and winning their due.

STILL SPEAKING FROM
SOMEWHERE IN PARTICULAR

I began this book by saying that each of us comes to ethical debates from somewhere in particular, and I acknowledged some of the particulars of my own life that influenced my feelings and reasons concerning Prozac and other forms of technologically shaping our selves. Much of this book has been to suggest that our own experience has everything to do with the stances and lenses to which we are partial and with the reasons that seem most salient to us. As quickly as possible, though, I stopped talking explicitly about any of the particulars of my experience. But I do not want to forget the words of Kay Redfield Jamison that I invoked in the beginning. "One is what one is, and the dishonesty of hiding behind a degree, or a title, or any manner and collection of words is still exactly that: dishonesty." I would fail to live up to the exhortation in her words and would fail to acknowledge the partiality of the view I have articulated, if I said nothing more about my experience since the early days of my involvement in these debates.

Alas, even though my personal and work lives are infinitely better than in the early days of my involvement in these debates, I still live with the same predispositions that made me accept that I should try to use medication when I was teaching in the lovely little town in Indiana that I mentioned in chapter 1. Today, to try to shape the features of my being that are difficult for me and for those closest to me, I use a variety of methods, including exercise, meditation, psychotherapy, and, yes, medication. It took me many years of struggling after my initial use of medication to be persuaded that I should try it again. I still dislike taking medication, not only because of the side effects I experience now and fear I will experience in the future, nor only because I don't want to be complicit with the medical-industrial complex or with the dominant norms of the society in which that complex is entrenched, but because of the difficult-to-shake feeling that using medication is a sign of moral weakness. At the moment I am writing, however—and the facts may change tomorrow—medication seems to make it a little easier to employ the other methods on that list. At the moment at least, it seems to help allow me to pursue the sorts of engagement with others and the world that I most want. For now, I think I flourish more with it than without it.

In the beginning of this book I acknowledged the respect in which the arguments I made against pharmacological "enhancement" early in my career were fueled by more than reason alone. Partly they were fueled by my desire to have and to exhibit the moral courage to stand up and say, No! Partly they were fueled by my deeply felt intuition regarding the ethical stance that we should take toward our selves and the world. Insofar as that intuition regarding the importance of letting things be is an essential component of my way of being in the world, those arguments were fueled in part by my desire to justify my way of being.

As you may now suspect, even if you lack formal psychiatric training, those arguments against pharmacological enhancement in general were also entangled with, and partly fueled by, my resistance to the idea of my own pharmacological treatment. It was easy to slip from imagining that I had justified a rejection of Prozac as a form of enhancement in general, to imagining that I had justified a rejection of it as a treatment for myself. In this way, too, my arguments back then were driven at least as much by my desire to justify my at-the-time *un*medicated way of being as by any impartial appraisal from reason alone.

I have just given you one more reason to suspect that the central point of this book—concerning the value of noticing the partiality of our insights and of embracing more binocular thinking—is also driven by more than reason alone. It is fueled not only by my insights, but also by my intuitions, and, of course, by my desire to justify my at-the-moment medicated way of being. I don't think there is a way for me to escape that truth about the ways in which my understanding is constrained. My guess, though, is that, no matter how marvelous your genome, childhood, and education, your thinking is constrained in your own way, too. I don't think we can escape such constraints, though I do think it can deepen our comprehension to become better at recognizing their presence.

One of the marvelous things about the field of bioethics in general, and about the technologically shaping our selves debates in particular, is that they invite us to ask the sorts of meaning questions that even a child can ask and that most adults, when given the chance, want to ask—no matter how impatient our societies have become with asking them. Bioethics in general and these debates in particular require us to step away from the pursuit of physical health and money and to ask what human flourishing entails. In the process of asking that question and the myriad meaning questions linked to it, we have the opportunity to be impressed by our capacity to give and take reasons that we hope can be understood by all. We also have the opportunity to be humbled by recognizing that the reasons we give always come from somewhere in particular. That recognition can help us deepen our comprehension, by prompting us to look from stances and through lenses that we are by nature and nurture less partial to. Asking meaning questions gives us the chance both to embrace rather than suppress the partiality of our insights and to do the same with the insights of others.

A second marvelous thing about bioethics in general, and about the debates concerning technologically shaping our selves in particular, is that they require us to answer practical ethical questions. They require us to garner confidence in the depth of our comprehension of what our own flourishing consists in and sometimes, far more rarely, to have confidence in the depth of our comprehension of what flourishing consists in for others. They require us to accept that, even though there are no final answers to the meaning questions that are always in the background of the practical ones, living a decent human life requires us to answer practical questions. They require us to accept that, just as our insights are ineluctably partial, so, too, are our answers.

It is easy to say that our insights and answers are partial and that a more binocular habit of thinking would deepen our comprehension of what's at stake in the debates about technologically shaping our selves. It is much harder to talk together as if we really grasped those simple facts. Perhaps this book can help someone who is new to these debates to grasp them more firmly than I did when I started out. If it could be of use to someone engaged in quite different debates, that would be all the more gratifying.

NOTES

Chapter 1

1. Daniel Callahan, *In Search of the Good Life: A Life in Bioethics* (New York: Cambridge University Press, 2012).
2. Cited in Susan E. Lederer, *Subjected to Science: Human Experimentation in America before the Second World War* (Baltimore, Md.: Johns Hopkins University Press, 1995), 1.
3. Willard Gaylin et al., *Doing Good: The Limits of Benevolence* (New York: Pantheon, 1978).
4. Cf. Lisa A. Eckenwiler and Felicia G. Cohn, eds., *The Ethics of Bioethics: Mapping the Moral Landscape* (Baltimore, Md.: Johns Hopkins University Press, 2007).
5. Toulmin Stephen, "How Medicine Saved the Life of Ethics," *Perspectives in Biology and Medicine* 25, no. 4 (1982): 736–50.
6. David H. Smith, "Stuck in the Middle," *Hastings Center Report* 36, no. 1 (2006): 32–33.
7. Milan Kundera, *The Unbearable Lightness of Being* (New York: Harper and Row, 1984), 139.
8. Ibid.
9. Kay Redfield Jamison, *An Unquiet Mind: A Memoir of Moods And Madness*, 1st ed. (New York: Vintage, 1995), 7.
10. Peter D. Kramer, *Listening to Prozac* (New York: Viking, 2005).
11. Walters published the key idea from that lecture a few years later. See LeRoy Walters and Julie Gage Palmer, "Enhancing Genetic Engineering," in *The*

Ethics of Human Gene Therapy (New York: Oxford University Press, 1997), 99–142.

12. Eric Juengst, "What Does Enhancement Mean?" in *Enhancing Human Traits: Ethical and Social Implications,* ed. Erik Parens (Washington, D.C.: Georgetown University Press, 1998), 29–47.

13. Anita Silvers, "A Fatal Attraction to Normalizing: Treating Disabilities as Deviations from 'Species-Typical' Functioning," in *Enhancing Human Traits: Ethical and Social Implications,* ed. Erik Parens (Washington, D.C.: Georgetown University Press, 1998), 95–123; Jackie Leach Scully and Christoph Rehmann-Sutter, "When Norms Normalize: The Case of Genetic 'Enhancement,'" *Human Gene Therapy* 12 (2001): 87–95.

14. Mark J. Hanson and Daniel Callahan, eds., *The Goals of Medicine: The Forgotten Issue in Health Care Reform* (Washington, D.C.: Georgetown University Press, 1999).

15. Erik Parens, "Is Enhancement Always Good? The Enhancement Project," *Hastings Center Report* 28, no. 1 (2012): S1–S17.

16. Daniel Kelly, *Yuck? The Nature and Moral Significance of Disgust* (Cambridge, Mass.: MIT Press, 2011).

17. Joshua Greene, *Moral Tribes: Emotion, Reason, and the Gap between Us and Them* (New York: Penguin, 2013).

18. Harriet McBryde Johnson, "Unspeakable Conversations," *New York Times,* February 16, 1993.

19. Adrienne Asch and Dorit Barlevy, "Disability and Genetics: A Disability Critique of Pre-Natal Testing and Preimplantation Genetic Diagnosis (PGD)," *eLS,* doi: 10.1002/9780470015902.a0005212.pub2

20. Julian Savulescu, "Procreative Beneficence: Why We Should Select the Best Children," *Bioethics* 15, no. 5–6 (2001): 413–26.

21. Derek A. Parfit, *Reasons and Persons* (Oxford: Oxford University Press, 1984).

22. Melinda A. Roberts and David T. Wasserman, eds., *Harming Future Persons: Ethics, Genetics and the Nonidentity Problem,* 1st ed. (New York: Springer, 2009).

23. Peter Singer, "Ethics and Institutions," *Journal of Ethics* 9 (2005): 331–52, at 349.

24. Ibid., 351.

25. Antonio Damasio, *Descartes' Error: Emotion, Reason, and the Human Brain* (New York: G. P. Putnam's Sons, 1994).

26. Martha C. Nussbaum, *Hiding from Humanity: Disgust, Shame, and the Law* (Princeton: Princeton University Press, 2004), chapter 2 (71–123).

27. Ibid., 109.

28. Erik Parens, *Enhancing Human Traits: Ethical and Social Implications* (Washington, D.C.: Georgetown University Press, 1998).

Chapter 2

1. Mihail C. Roco and William Sims Bainbridge, eds., *Converging Technologies for Improving Human Performance: Nanotechnology, Biotechnology, Information Technology and Cognitive Science* (Dordrecht: Kluwer Academic, 2003).
2. Peter D. Kramer, *Listening to Prozac* (New York: Viking, 2005).
3. Cassandra Aspinall, "Do I Make You Uncomfortable? Reflections on Using Surgery to Reduce the Distress of Others," in *Surgically Shaping Children: Technology, Ethics, and the Pursuit of Normality*, ed. Erik Parens (Baltimore, Md.: Johns Hopkins University Press, 2006), 13–28.
4. Carl Elliott, *Better Than Well: American Medicine Meets the American Dream* (New York: W. W. Norton, 2003).
5. Nicholas Agar, *Humanity's End: Why We Should Reject Radical Enhancement* (Cambridge, Mass.: MIT Press, 2010).
6. Victoria Pitts, *In the Flesh: The Cultural Politics of Body Modification* (New York: Palgrave Macmillan, 2003).
7. Jonathan Glover, "Towards Humanism in Psychiatry," *Tanner Lectures on Human Values* (2003): 511–52, at 551.
8. Jonathan Glover, *Choosing Children: Genes, Disability, and Design* (New York: Oxford University Press, 2006), 93–95.
9. Thomas Nagel, "What Is It Like to Be a Bat?" *Philosophical Review* 83, no. 4 (1974): 435–50.
10. Wilhelm Dilthey, "Introduction to the Human Sciences," in *Wilhelm Dilthey: Selected Works, Vol. 1*, ed. Rudolf Makkreel and Frithjof Rodi (Princeton, N.J.: Princeton University Press, 1989).
11. Hans Jonas, *The Phenomenon of Life: Toward Philosophical Biology* (Chicago: University of Chicago Press, 1966).
12. Jacques Derrida, "Structure, Sign, and Play," in *Writing and Difference*, trans. Alan Bass (Chicago: University of Chicago Press, 1978), 280–81.
13. Ludwig Wittgenstein, *Philosophical Investigations*, trans. G. E. M. Anscombe (New York: Macmillan, 1953), 194ᵉ.
14. Cited in Jonathan Haidt, *The Righteous Mind: Why Good People Are Divided by Politics and Religion* (New York: Pantheon, 2012), xvii.

Chapter 3

1. Leon Kass, "The Wisdom of Repugnance," *New Republic* (June 2, 1997): 17–26.
2. Yuval Levin, *Imagining the Future: Science and American Democracy* (New York: Encounter, 2008).

3. John Harris, *Enhancing Evolution: The Ethical Case for Making Better People* (Princeton, N.J.: Princeton University Press, 2007).

4. Michael Henry, Jennifer R. Fishman, and Stuart J. Youngner, "Propranolol and the Prevention of Post-traumatic Stress Disorder: Is It Wrong to Erase the 'Sting' of Bad Memories?" *American Journal of Bioethics* 7, no. 9 (September 2007): 12–20, http://www.ncbi.nlm.nih.gov/pubmed/17849331.

5. Charles Taylor, *Sources of the Self: The Making of the Modern Identity* (Cambridge, Mass.: Harvard University Press, 1989).

6. Charles Taylor, *The Ethics of Authenticity* (Cambridge, Mass.: Harvard University Press, 1991).

7. Ibid., 29.

8. Ibid., 18.

9. Ibid., 16.

10. Ibid., 17.

11. Ibid., 17–18.

12. Carl Elliott and Tod Chambers, eds., *Prozac as a Way of Life* (Chapel Hill: University of North Carolina Press, 2004); Carl Elliott, *Better Than Well: American Medicine Meets the American Dream* (New York: W. W. Norton, 2003); Carl Elliott, "The Tyranny of Happiness: Ethics and Cosmetic Psychopharmacology," in *Enhancing Human Traits: Ethical and Social Implications*, ed. Erik Parens (Washington, D.C.: Georgetown University Press, 1998), 177–88.

13. Neil Levy, "Enhancing Authenticity," *Journal of Applied Philosophy* 28, no. 3 (August 7, 2011): 308–18.

14. Neil Levy, *Neuroethics: Challenges for the 21st Century* (Cambridge: Cambridge University Press, 2007).

15. Taylor, *Ethics of Authenticity*, 73.

16. President's Council on Bioethics, *Beyond Therapy: Biotechnology and the Pursuit of Happiness*, 1st ed. (New York: HarperCollins, 2003).

17. Ibid., 294.

18. Allen Buchanan, *Beyond Humanity?* (New York: Oxford University Press, 2011).

19. Levin, *Imagining the Future*.

20. James Hughes, *Citizen Cyborg* (Cambridge, Mass.: Westview, 2004).

21. Susan Bordo, *Unbearable Weight: Feminism, Western Culture, and the Body* (Berkeley: University of California Press, 1993); Alice Dreger, *One of Us: Conjoined Twins and the Future of Normal* (Cambridge, Mass.: Harvard University Press, 2004); Rob Sparrow, "Liberalism and Eugenics," *Australasian Journal of Philosophy* 89, no. 3 (2010): 499–517, doi: 10.1080/00 048402.2010.484464; Michael Hauskeller, *Better Humans? Understanding the Enhancement Project* (Durham, U.K.: Acumen, 2013).

22. Elliott, *Better Than Well*.

23. Ibid., 16.
24. Elliott, "Tyranny of Happiness."
25. Ibid., 180.
26. Walker Percy, *The Moviegoer* (New York: Random House, 1998).
27. Epigraph to Percy, *Moviegoer*. See also Søren Kierkegaard, *The Sickness Unto Death*, trans. Alastair Hannay (London: Penguin, 1989 [1849]), 75.
28. Peter D. Kramer, *Listening to Prozac* (New York: Viking, 2005), 258.
29. David DeGrazia, "Prozac, Enhancement, and Self-Creation," in *Prozac as a Way of Life*, ed. Carl Elliott and Tod Chambers (Chapel Hill: University of North Carolina Press, 2004), 33–47. See also David DeGrazia, *Bioethics and Human Identity* (New York: Cambridge University Press, 2009).
30. DeGrazia, "Prozac, Enhancement, and Self-Creation," 41.
31. Harlan Lane, *When the Mind Hears: A History of the Deaf* (New York: Random House, 1984); Robert A. Crouch, "Letting the Deaf Be Deaf: Reconsidering the Use of Cochlear Implants in Prelingually Deaf Children," *Hastings Center Report* (1997): 14–21.
32. Michael Chorost, *Rebuilt: How Becoming Part Computer Made Me More Human* (New York: Houghton Mifflin, 2005), 188.
33. Ibid., 195.
34. Kathy Davis, *Reshaping the Female Body: The Dilemma of Cosmetic Surgery* (New York: Routledge, 1995).
35. Ibid., 77.
36. Ilina Singh, "Not Robots: Children's Perspectives on Authenticity, Moral Agency and Stimulant Drug Treatments," *Journal of Medical Ethics* (August 28, 2012): 1–8, http://www.ncbi.nlm.nih.gov/pubmed/22930677.
37. Richard M. Berlin, ed., *Poets on Prozac: Mental Illness, Treatment, and the Creative Process* (Baltimore, Md.: Johns Hopkins University Press, 2008).
38. Tony Hope et al., "Anorexia Nervosa and the Language of Authenticity," *Hastings Center Report* (2011): 1–10.
39. Josephine Johnston and Carl Elliott, "Healthy Limb Amputation: Ethical and Legal Aspects," *Clinical Medicine* 2, no. 5 (October 2002): 431–35, http://www.ncbi.nlm.nih.gov/pubmed/12448590.
40. Melody Gilbert, *Whole: A Documentary* (FRZN Productions, 2003).
41. Janice G. Raymond, *The Transsexual Empire: The Making of the She-Male* (New York: Teachers College Press, 1979).
42. Jamison Green, *Becoming a Visible Man* (Nashville, Tenn.: Vanderbilt University Press, 2004).
43. Hughes, *Citizen Cyborg*.
44. Michael Sandel, *The Case against Perfection* (Cambridge, Mass.: Belknap Press of Harvard University Press, 2007), 29.
45. Ibid., 45.
46. Levy, *Neuroethics*, xiii.

47. Sandel, *Case against Perfection*, 27.
48. Michael Hauskeller, "Human Enhancement and the Giftedness of Life," *Philosophical Papers* 40, no. 1 (2011): 55–79, at 77.
49. Jackie Leach Scully, Tom Shakespeare, and Sarah Banks, "Gift or Commodity? Lay People Deliberating Social Sex Selection," *Sociology of Health and Illness* 28, no. 6 (2006): 749–67.
50. Richard Dawkins, The God Delusion (London: Bantam, 2006); Daniel Dennett, Breaking the Spell: Religion as a Natural Phenomenon (New York: Penguin, 2006); Sam Harris, The End of Faith: Religion, Terror, and the Future of Reason (New York: W. W. Norton, 2005); Christopher Hitchens, God Is Not Great: How Religion Poisons Everything (New York: Hachette, 2007).
51. Buchanan, *Beyond Humanity?*
52. Paul Ramsey, *Fabricated Man: The Ethics of Genetic Control* (New Haven, Conn.: Yale University Press, 1970).
53. Joseph Fletcher, *The Ethics of Genetic Control* (Buffalo, N.Y.: Prometheus, 1988).
54. Julian Savulescu, Bennett Foddy, and Megan Clayton, "Why We Should Allow Performance Enhancing Drugs in Sport: Human Enhancement and the Human Spirit," *British Journal of Sports Medicine* 38, no. 6 (2004): 666–75, at 667.
55. Thomas H. Murray, *The Worth of a Child* (Berkeley: University of California Press, 1996).
56. Ibid., 136.
57. Hans Jonas, "The Burden and Blessing of Mortality," *Hastings Center Report* 22, no. 1 (1992): 36.
58. Joshua Wolf Shenk, *Lincoln's Melancholy: How Depression Challenged a President and Fueled His Greatness* (New York: Houghton Mifflin, 2005).
59. Bruce Jennings, "Enlightenment and Enchantment: Technology and Moral Limits," *Technology in Society* 32 (2010): 25–30.
60. David Pearce, "The Hedonistic Imperative," n.d., http://www.hedweb.com/.
61. Peter Kramer, *Against Depression* (New York: Penguin, 2005).
62. Buchanan, *Beyond Humanity?*
63. Chris Zarpentine, "The Thorny and Arduous Path of Moral Progress: Moral Psychology and Moral Enhancement," *Neuroethics* 6 (2013): 141–53.

Chapter 4

1. Erik Parens, "Is Better Always Good?" 1–28, and Ronald Cole Turner, "Do Means Matter?" 151–61, both in *Enhancing Human Traits*, ed. Erik Parens (Washington, D.C.: Georgetown University Press, 1998).

2. Hilary Putnam, *The Collapse of the Fact/Value Dichotomy* (Cambridge, Mass.: Harvard University Press, 2002), 63.

3. Philip Ball, *Unnatural: The Heretical Idea of Making People* (London: Bodley Head, Random House, 2011).

4. *Splicing Life: A Report on the Social and Ethical Issues of Genetic Engineering with Human Beings* (Washington, D.C., 1982), 31.

5. Robert Carlson, *Biology Is Technology* (Cambridge, Mass.: Harvard University Press, 2010), 1.

6. Dan Brock, "Enhancement of Human Function: Some Distinctions for Policy Makers," in *Enhancing Human Traits*, ed. Erik Parens (Washington, D.C.: Georgetown University Press, 1998), 48–69.

7. For an updated version of such optimism, see S. Matthew Liao, Anders Sandberg, and Rebecca Roache, "Human Engineering and Climate Change," *Ethics, Policy and Environment* 15, no. 2 (2012): 206–21.

8. Jacob Moses, "The 1.5 Cultures Problem," *Hastings Center Report* 41, no. 6 (2011): inside front cover.

9. David Hume, *A Treatise of Human Nature*, Book III, Part 1, Section 1 (London: Penguin, 1985), 521.

10. Donna J. Haraway, *Simians, Cyborgs, and Women: The Reinvention of Nature* (New York: Routledge, 1991).

11. Andy Clark, *Natural-Born Cyborgs* (New York: Oxford University Press, 2003).

12. Andy Clark and David Chalmers, "The Extended Mind," *Analysis* 58 (1998): 10–23.

13. Ibid., 8.

14. Neil Levy, *Neuroethics: Challenges for the 21st Century* (Cambridge, U.K.: Cambridge University Press, 2007).

15. John Stuart Mill, "Nature," in *Essential Works of John Stuart Mill* (New York: Bantam, 1961), 361–401, at 401.

16. Or, as Langdon Winner once put it, "artifacts have politics." See *The Whale and the Reactor: A Search for Limits in an Age of High Technology* (Chicago: University of Chicago Press, 1986).

17. James C. Edwards, "Concepts of Technology and Their Role in Moral Reflection," in *Surgically Shaping Children: Technology, Ethics, and the Pursuit of Normality*, ed. Erik Parens (Baltimore, Md.: Johns Hopkins University Press, 2006), 51–67, at 55.

18. Dena Davis, *Genetic Dilemmas: Reproductive Technology, Parental Choices, and Children's Futures* (New York: Routledge, 2001).

19. Michael Berube, *Life as We Know It* (New York: Pantheon, 1996); Nancy Press, "Assessing the Expressive Character of Prenatal Testing: The Choices Made or the Choices Made Available?" in *Prenatal Testing and Disability Rights*, ed. Erik Parens and Adrienne Asch (Washington, D.C.: Georgetown University Press, 2000), 214–33.

20. Barbara A. Koenig, "The Technological Imperative in Medical Practice: The Social Creation of a 'Routine' Treatment," in *Biomedicine Reexamined*, ed. Margaret Lock and Deborah R. Gordon (Dordrecht, the Netherlands: Kluwer Academic, 1998), 465–96.
21. Edwards, "Concepts of Technology."
22. Ibid.
23. Leslie C. Aiello and Peter Wheeler, "The Expensive-Tissue Hypothesis: The Brain and the Digestive System in Human and Primate Evolution," *Current Anthropology* 36, no. 2 (1995): 199–221.
24. Russell Blackford, "Sinning against Nature: The Theory of Background Conditions," *Journal of Medical Ethics* 32 (2006): 629–34.
25. "BP's Oil Leak in the Gulf Is a 'Natural Disaster,' Just Like BP's Public Relations Efforts," *Comedy Central*, June 30, 2010, http://www.indecisionfor ever.com/blog/2010/06/30/bps-oil-leak-in-the-gulf-is-a-natural-disaster-just-like-bps-public-relations-efforts.
26. Bob Herbert, "An Unnatural Disaster," *New York Times*, May 28, 2010.
27. Nick Bostrom and Toby Ord, "The Reversal Test: Eliminating Status Quo Bias in Applied Ethics," *Ethics* 116 (2006): 656–79.
28. For example, Ray Kurzweil, *The Singularity Is Near: When Humans Transcend Biology* (New York: Viking, 2005).
29. Albert Borgmann, *Technology and the Character of Contemporary Life: A Philosophical Inquiry* (Chicago: University of Chicago Press, 1984), 221.
30. Maartje Schermer, "Enhancements, Easy Shortcuts, and the Richness of Human Activities," *Bioethics* 22, no. 7 (August 2008): 355–63.
31. John Stuart Mill, *On Liberty*, ed. Elizabeth Rapaport (Indianapolis, Ind.: Hackett, 1978 [1859]), 54.

Chapter 5

1. James Hughes, *Citizen Cyborg* (Cambridge, Mass.: Westview, 2004), 205.
2. Robert Nozick, *Anarchy, State, and Utopia* (New York: Basic, 1974), 42–45.
3. Felipe De Brigard, "If You Like It, Does It Matter If It's Real?" *Philosophical Psychology* 23, no. 1 (1020): 43–57.
4. Jonathan Glover, *Choosing Children: Genes, Disability, and Design* (New York: Oxford University Press, 2006), 91.
5. President's Council on Bioethics, *Beyond Therapy: Biotechnology and the Pursuit of Happiness* (New York: HarperCollins, 2003), 253.
6. Ibid.
7. John Harris, *Enhancing Evolution: The Ethical Case for Making Better People* (Princeton, N.J.: Princeton University Press, 2007), 153.
8. Julian Savulescu and Anders Sandberg, "Neuroenhancement of Love and Marriage: The Chemicals between Us," *Neuroethics* 1, no. 1 (2008): 31–44.

9. Harris, *Enhancing Evolution*, 136.

10. Saskia K. Nagel, *Ethics and the Neurosciences* (Paderborn, Germany: Mentis, 2010), 214.

11. Ibid., 208.

12. Allen Buchanan, *Beyond Humanity?* (New York: Oxford University Press, 2011), 16.

13. Francis Fukuyama, *Our Posthuman Future* (New York: Farrar, Straus & Giroux, 2002).

14. Leon R. Kass, "The Wisdom of Repugnance," *The New Republic* (June 2, 1997): 17–26.

15. Jürgen Habermas, *The Future of Human Nature* (Malden, Mass.: Polity, 2003).

16. Fukuyama, *Our Posthuman Future*, 183.

17. President's Council on Bioethics, *Beyond Therapy*, 310.

18. Michael Henry, Jennifer R. Fishman, and Stuart J. Youngner, "Propranolol and the Prevention of Post-traumatic Stress Disorder: Is It Wrong to Erase the 'Sting' of Bad Memories?" *American Journal of Bioethics* 7, no. 9 (2007): 12–20, at 17, http://www.ncbi.nlm.nih.gov/pubmed/17849331.

19. See Neil Levy, *Neuroethics: Challenges for the 21st Century* (Cambridge: Cambridge University Press, 2007), 171–72; David Wasserman, "Making Memory Lose Its Sting," *Philosophy and Public Policy Quarterly* 4, no. 4 (2004): 12–18, at 13.

20. Henry, Fishman, and Youngner, "Propranolol and the Prevention of Post-traumatic Stress Disorder," 14.

21. President's Council on Bioethics, *Beyond Therapy*, 225.

22. Peter Conrad, *The Medicalization of Society* (Baltimore, Md.: Johns Hopkins University Press, 2007).

23. Henry, Fishman, and Youngner, "Propranolol and the Prevention of Post-traumatic Stress Disorder," 18.

24. P. Alex Linley and Stephen Joseph, "Positive Change Following Trauma and Adversity: A Review," *Journal of Traumatic Stress* 17, no. 1 (2004): 11–21.

25. President's Council on Bioethics, *Beyond Therapy*, 220.

26. Ibid., 226.

27. Deane Aikens, "The Use of Pharmacology to Augment Psychotherapy Gains," unpublished manuscript.

28. Sigmund Freud, *Civilization and Its Discontents* (New York: W. W. Norton, 1961), 61.

Chapter 6

1. Thomas Nagel, "What Is It Like to Be a Bat?" *Philosophical Review* 83, no. 4 (1974): 435–50.

2. Carl Schoonover, ed., *Portraits of the Mind* (New York: Abrams, 2010).

3. Jonah Lehrer, "Foreword," in Carl Schoonover, ed., *Portraits of the Mind* (New York: Abrams, 2010), 6–7, at 6.

4. Joy Hirsch, "From Brain Structure to Brain Function," in Carl Schoonover, ed., *Portraits of the Mind* (New York: Abrams, 2010), 200–225.

5. Francis Crick, *The Astonishing Hypothesis: The Scientific Search for the Soul* (New York: Touchstone, 1994).

6. Christof Koch, *The Quest for Consciousness* (Englewood, Colo.: Roberts and Company, 2004).

7. Crick, *The Astonishing Hypothesis*, 3.

8. Walter G1lannon, "Our Brains Are Not Us," in *Brain, Body, and Mind: Neuroethics with a Human Face* (New York: Oxford University Press, 2011), 11–40.

9. Joshua Greene and Jonathan Cohen, "For the Law, Neuroscience Changes Nothing and Everything," *Philosophical Transactions of the Royal Society of London. Series B, Biological Sciences* 359 (2004): 1775–85; Sam Harris, *Free Will* (New York: Simon and Schuster, 2012); Daniel Wegner, *The Illusion of Conscious Will* (Cambridge, Mass.: MIT Press, 2002).

10. Crick, *The Astonishing Hypothesis*, 31.

11. Daniel Dennett, "Explaining the 'Magic' of Consciousness," *Journal of Cultural and Evolutionary Psychology* 1, no. 1 (2003): 7–19.

12. Paul Ricoeur, *Freud and Philosophy: An Essay on Interpretation* (New Haven, Conn.: Yale University Press, 1977).

13. Hans Jonas, *The Phenomenon of Life: Toward a Philosophical Biology* (Chicago: University of Chicago Press, 1966); Leon Kass, *Toward a More Natural Science: Biology and Human Affairs* (New York: Free Press, 1985); Gerald McKenny, *To Relieve the Human Condition: Bioethics, Technology, and the Body* (Albany, N.Y.: SUNY Press, 1997).

14. Alva Noë, *Out of Our Heads: Why You Are Not Your Brain, and Other Lessons of the Biology of Consciousness* (New York: Hill and Wang, 2009).

15. Ibid., 140.

16. Ibid., 142.

Chapter 7

1. Michael Oliver, *Social Work with Disabled People* (Basingstoke, U.K.: Macmillan, 1983).

2. Nora Ellen Groce, *Everyone Here Spoke Sign Language* (Cambridge, Mass.: Harvard University Press, 1985).

3. Tom Shakespeare, *Disability Rights and Wrongs* (New York: Routledge, 2006).

4. Jackie Leach Scully, *Disability Bioethics: Moral Bodies, Moral Difference* (Lanham, Md.: Rowman and Littlefield, 2008).

5. Phillip V. Davis and John G. Bradley, "The Meaning of Normal," *Perspectives in Biology and Medicine* 40, no. 1 (1996): 68–77.

6. Eva Feder Kittay, "Thoughts on the Desire for Normality," in *Surgically Shaping Children: Technology, Ethics, and the Pursuit of Normality*, ed. Erik Parens (Baltimore, Md.: Johns Hopkins University Press, 2006), 90–112.

7. Lisa Abelow Hedley, "The Seduction of the Surgical Fix," in *Surgically Shaping Children: Technology, Ethics, and the Pursuit of Normality*, ed. Erik Parens (Baltimore, Md.: Johns Hopkins University Press, 2006), 43–50.

8. William F. May, "The President's Council on Bioethics," *Perspectives in Biology and Medicine* 48, no. 2 (2005): 229–40; Michael Sandel, *The Case against Perfection* (Cambridge, Mass.: Belknap Press of Harvard University Press, 2007); Ronald M. Green, *Babies by Design* (New Haven, Conn.: Yale University Press, 2008); Dov Fox, "Parental Attention Deficit Disorder," *Journal of Applied Philosophy* 25, no. 3 (2008): 246–61.

9. Alice Domurat Dreger, *Hermaphrodites and the Medical Invention of Sex* (Cambridge, Mass.: Harvard University Press, 1998).

10. Alice Donurat Dreger, ed., *Intersex in the Age of Ethics* (Frederick, Md.: University Publishing Group, 1999).

11. Cassandra Aspinall, "Do I Make You Uncomfortable? Reflections on Using Surgery to Reduce the Distress of Others," in *Surgically Shaping Children: Technology, Ethics, and the Pursuit of Normality*, ed. Erik Parens (Baltimore, Md.: Johns Hopkins University Press, 2006), 13–28.

12. Emily Sullivan Sanford, "My Shoe Size Stayed the Same: Maintaining a Positive Sense of Identity with Achondroplasia and Limb-Lengthening Surgeries," in *Surgically Shaping Children: Technology, Ethics, and the Pursuit of Normality*, ed. Erik Parens (Baltimore, Md.: Johns Hopkins University Press, 2006), 29–43.

13. Hilde Lindemann Nelson and James Lindemann Nelson, *The Patient in the Family: An Ethics of Medicine and Families* (New York: Routledge, 1995); Thomas Murray, *The Worth of a Child* (Berkeley: University of California Press, 1996).

14. Committee on Bioethics, "Informed Consent, Parental Permission, and Assent in Pediatric Practice," *Pediatrics* 95, no. 2 (2012): 314–17.

15. Adrienne Asch, "Appearance-Altering Surgery, Children's Sense of Self, and Parental Love," in *Surgically Shaping Children: Technology, Ethics, and the Pursuit of Normality*, ed. Erik Parens (Baltimore, Md.: Johns Hopkins University Press, 2006), 227–52.

16. This child was a patient in Cassandra Aspinall's craniofacial clinic, and she gave permission for me to use this information.

17. Asch, "Appearance-Altering Surgery," 239.

18. Gary L. Albrecht and Patrick J. Devlieger, "The Disability Paradox: High Quality of Life against All Odds," *Social Science and Medicine* 48, no. 8 (1999): 977–88.

19. Saroj Saigal et al., "Differences in Preferences for Neonatal Outcomes among Health Care Professionals, Parents, and Adolescents," *Journal of the American Medical Association* 281, no. 21 (1999): 1991–97.

20. Jason Riis et al., "Ignorance of Hedonic Adaptation to Hemodialysis: A Study Using Ecological Momentary Assessment," *Journal of Experimental Psychology* 134, no. 1 (2005): 3–9.

21. Peter A. Ubel et al., "Misimagining the Unimaginable: The Disability Paradox and Health Care Decision Making," *Health Psychology* 24, no. 4 (2005): 57–62.

22. Sunil Kothari and Kristi Kirschner, "Abandoning the Golden Rule: The Problem with Putting Ourselves in the Patient's Place," *Topics in Stroke Rehabilitation* 13, no. 4 (2006): 66–73.

23. Imelda Coyne and Pamela Gallagher, "Participation in Communication and Decision-Making: Children and Young People's Experiences in a Hospital Setting," *Journal of Clinical Nursing* 20 (2011): 2334–43.

24. Priscilla Alderson, *Children's Consent to Surgery* (Buckingham, U.K.: Open University Press, 1993).

25. Isaiah Berlin, "The Pursuit of the Ideal," in *The Crooked Timber of Humanity*, ed. Henry Hardy (New York: Vintage, 1959, 1992), 1–19, at 19.

Closing Thoughts

1. Antonio R. Damasio, *Descartes' Error: Emotion, Reason, and the Human Brain* (New York: G. P. Putnam's Sons, 1994).

2. Lawrence Kohlberg, "Stage and Sequence: The Cognitive-Developmental Approach to Socialization," in *Handbook of Socialization Theory and Research*, ed. David A. Goslin (Chicago: Rand McNally, 1969), 347–480.

3. Jonathan Haidt, "The Emotional Dog and Its Rational Tail: A Social Intuitionist Approach to Moral Judgment," *Psychological Review* 108, no. 4 (2001): 814–34.

4. John Searle, *Mind: A Brief Introduction* (Oxford: Oxford University Press, 2004), 135.

5. Isaiah Berlin, "The Pursuit of the Ideal," in *The Crooked Timber of Humanity*, ed. Henry Hardy (New York: Vintage, [1959]/1992); Martha Nussbaum, "Non-relative Virtues: An Aristotelian Approach," in *The Quality of Life*, ed. Martha Nussbaum and Amartya Sen (New York: Oxford University Press, 1983), 242–69; Amy Gutmann, "The Challenge of Multiculturalism in Political Ethics," *Philosophy and Public Affairs* 22 (1993): 171–206; Jonathan Glover, *Choosing Children: Genes, Disability, and Design* (New York: Oxford University Press, 2006), 93–95.

6. Cited in Hilary Putnam, "Fact and Value in the World of Amartya Sen," in *The Collapse of the Fact/Value Dichotomy and Other Essays* (Cambridge, Mass.: Harvard University Press, 2002), 69.

7. President's Council on Bioethics, *Beyond Therapy: Biotechnology and the Pursuit of Happiness* (New York: HarperCollins, 2003), 310; Neil Levy, *Neuroethics: Challenges for the 21st Century* (Cambridge: Cambridge University Press, 2007), 120.

8. Richard Wilkinson and Kate Pickett, *The Spirit Level: Why More Equal Societies Almost Always Do Better* (London: Allen Lane/Penguin, 2009); Joseph Stiglitz, Amartya Sen, and Jean-Paul Fitoussi, *Report by the Commission on the Measurement of Economic Performance and Social Progress* (2009), www.stiglitz-sen-fitoussi.fr.

9. Hugo Mercier and Dan Sperber, "Why Do Humans Reason? Arguments for an Argumentative Theory," *Behavioral and Brain Sciences* 34 (2011): 57–111, doi:10.1017/S0140525X10000968.

10. Buchanan, *Beyond Humanity?*

11. John Harris, "Ethics Is for Bad Guys! Putting the 'Moral' into Moral Enhancement," *Bioethics* (2012): 169–73.

12. James Hughes, "Contradictions from the Enlightenment Roots of Transhumanism," *Journal of Medicine and Philosophy* 35 (2010): 622–40.

INDEX

CPSIA information can be obtained at www.ICGtesting.com
Printed in the USA
BVOW08s1208240716

456330BV00002B/4/P